Fluids and Electrolytes

Second Edition

Fluids and Electrolytes

A Conceptual Approach

Second Edition

E. KINSEY M. SMITH, M.D. (Lond.),
F.R.C.P., F.R.C.P.(C)
Professor, Department of Medicine
and Associate Dean (Education)
Faculty of Health Sciences,
McMaster University
Hamilton, Ontario, Canada

Illustrated by:
David Lemmond
Audio Visual Services,
Faculty of Health Sciences
McMaster University
Hamilton, Ontario, Canada

Text preparation by:
Josie Di Nello
Nephrology Department,
St. Joseph's Hospital
Hamilton, Ontario, Canada

Churchill Livingstone
New York, Edinburgh, London, Melbourne, Tokyo

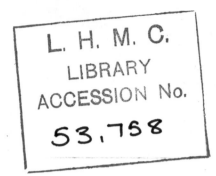
Library of Congress Cataloging-in-Publication Data

Smith, Kinsey.
    Fluids and electrolytes : a conceptual approach / E. Kinsey M.
Smith ; illustrated by David Lemmond ; text preparation by Josie Di
Nello. —2nd ed.
        p. cm
    Includes bibliographical references and index.
    ISBN 0-443-08796-2
    1. Body fluids. 2. Water-electrolyte balance (Physiology)
3. Body fluid disorders. 4. Water-electrolyte imbalances.
I. Title.
    [DNLM: 1. Body Fluids. 2. Water-Electrolyte Balance. QU 105
S435f]
QP90.5.S63 1991
612′.01522—dc20
DLC
for Library of Congress   91-10960
                                                              CIP

Second Edition © Churchill Livingstone Inc. 1991
First Edition © Churchill Livingstone Inc. 1980

Distributed in the United Kingdom by Churchill Livingstone, Robert Stevenson
House, 1–3 Baxter's Place, Leith Walk, Edinburgh EH1 3AF, and by associated
companies, branches, and representatives throughout the world.

Accurate indications, adverse reactions, and dosage schedules for drugs are provided in this book, but it is possible that they may change. The reader is urged to
review the package information data of the manufacturers of the medications mentioned.

The Publishers have made every effort to trace the copyright holders for borrowed
material. If they have inadvertently overlooked any, they will be pleased to make
the necessary arrangements at the first opportunity.

Printed in the United States of America

First published in 1991   7 6 5 4 3 2 1

To P.J.S.

Preface to the Second Edition

The second edition of this book follows the same format as its predecessor and its companion volume - "Renal Disease - A Conceptual Approach". Concepts have been emphasized and the problems faced by students with limited science background and the stress of a "packed curriculum" have been kept in mind. The illustrations are an essential complement to the text and in the first edition suffered from variability of style and quality. This has been corrected by the skill and imagination of David Lemmond using computer based technology.

The text has been revised, significant new knowledge has been incorporated and an index has been added. In spite of this, the book has not been increased in length, and it is hoped that this will avoid a sense of "information overload" at a time when more scholarly modern texts are often perceived to be intimidating because of their complexity and size. This book is complementary to such texts and should serve as an introduction to their use and not as a replacement for them.

I wish to thank the Audio Visual Department at McMaster who have provided superb resources, the students who continue to make academic life a happy challenge and my colleagues in the Faculty of Health Sciences who have supported my attempts to be an educator over the past two decades.

Kinsey Smith (1991)

Preface to the First Edition

This illustrated text was developed primarily for undergraduate medical students at McMaster University. Some of these students do not have any background in the physical or biological sciences, and many of the basic concepts they need for the understanding of body fluid regulation are foreign to them. Moreover, the constraints of a three year undergraduate course emphasize the value of clear introductory resources which link basic concepts to relevant clinical problems.

This book attempts to introduce the idea of a regulated internal environment and its responses in health and disease. The illustrations provide a visual summary, the text a simple and direct description of the illustrated concepts. It does not pretend to be comprehensive and the student should not use it to replace more detailed and scholarly resources. The method of presentation is not conventional, but the underlying concepts are well established and lean heavily upon the influence of other authors; the references provided at the end of the book represent only a small selection of useful resources and do no more than point the way to wider reading. The lucid writings of the late L.G. Welt and R.F. Pitts have been especially valuable to me and I make no apology for the major influence they have had in the development of the concepts that are illustrated here. Many ideas for visual presentation have come from the enthusiasm of Dr. Elizabeth Brain and members of the Audio Visual Department, and thanks are due to those colleagues amongst students and faculty who have provided stimulation and advice over the past decade.

This text is based in part upon material that has been used in a slide/tape format for a number of years. It is now offered to a wider readership in the hope that it may prove useful in other medical, nursing and paramedical programmes and perhaps as a reminder for more advanced students.

Kinsey Smith (1980)

Table of Contents

Table of Contents

Chapter 1

The Cellular Environment

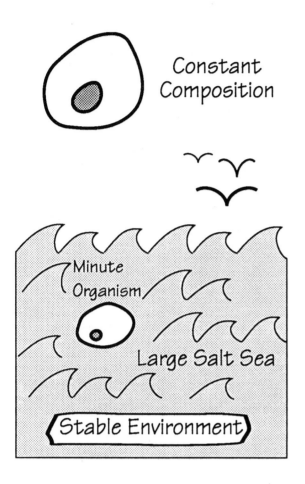

Constant Composition

Minute Organism

Large Salt Sea

Stable Environment

The Cell

The unit of biological function is the single cell which requires a defined composition to function normally. It must be capable of acquiring vital nutrients as they become depleted and of rejecting those end products which are not required and are potentially toxic.

...and its Surroundings

Simple, single-celled organisms evolving in an almost infinitely large salt sea may be considered as having an unvarying external environment. In this setting, regulation of their volume and composition is relatively simple. Surrounding osmotic pressures do not change appreciably and the concentration of solutes around them is constant. Waste products can simply diffuse out of the cell and become infinitely diluted in the surrounding sea.

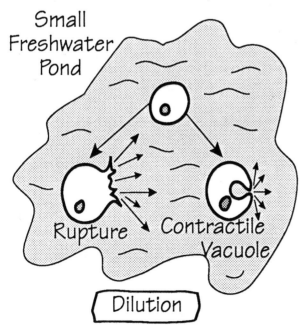

Small Freshwater Pond

Rupture Contractile Vacuole

Dilution

A single-celled organism (such as an ameba) living in a small fresh water pond faces a more hostile environment. A vigorous rain storm may dilute the already solute-poor water in the pond and produce increasing osmotic pressure gradients which cause water to enter the cell which will swell up to the point of bursting.

Adaptations which prevent this happening include the evolution of such devices as "contractile vacuoles" which can eject unwelcome volume.

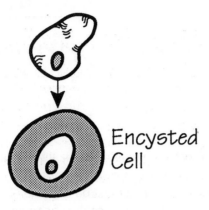

Encysted
Cell

If the pond dries up, the reverse process occurs and the cell becomes shrivelled and dehydrated. The protection such an organism can provide for itself is to become encysted, surrounding itself with a "waterproof coat" which will allow it to withstand desiccation and become reactivated when conditions improve. The price paid for this survival is to undergo periods of immobility and inactivity.

"The Milieu Interieur"

Warm blooded multicellular animals, like man, have adapted to life on dry land by taking with them a "personal environment", the composition and volume of which are precisely regulated even in the face of widely varying external conditions. This environment is like a "shell" of fluid which allows the cells to ignore changes in the outside world. This insulating shell is the "milieu interieur" (internal environment), first recognized by Claude Bernard and provided by the extracellular fluids.

In complex animals the body fluids can thus be separated into two compartments, the intracellular fluid (I.C.F.) and the extracellular fluid (E.C.F.).

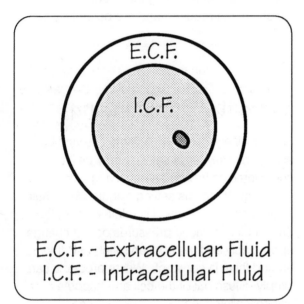

E.C.F.

I.C.F.

E.C.F. - Extracellular Fluid
I.C.F. - Intracellular Fluid

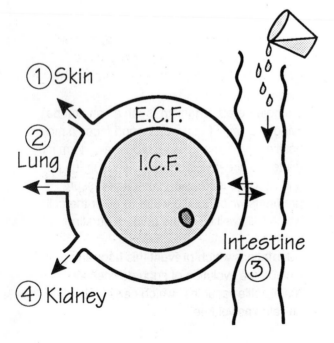

① Skin

② Lung

E.C.F.

I.C.F.

Intestine ③

④ Kidney

The only natural entry point to the body fluid compartments is by the mouth and intestinal tract. There are four exit routes from the extracellular fluid space and these are:

1) The skin, where loss occurs by perspiration and is related to temperature and humidity.

2) The lung, where loss is related to the need to moisten the air we breathe.

3) The intestine, where diarrhea or vomiting may cause abnormal losses.

4) The kidney, which is the only exit route that can be closely regulated.

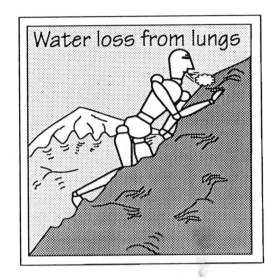

Fluid Loss from the E.C.F.

Losses via the skin and the lung are dependent upon external factors which cannot be controlled. Thus men climbing high mountains in cold, dry air will have enormous water losses from the lungs as hypoxia demands increased ventilation. In early attempts to climb Mount Everest the inability to carry enough fuel to melt enough snow to prevent dehydration was a major cause of failure.

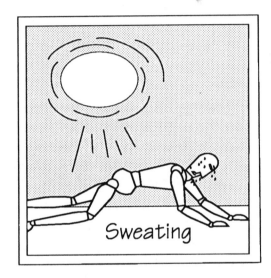

Men suddenly transported to a hot climate may sweat unmanageably and become dangerously volume deplete. Adaptation to such a climate takes a week or two and studies of troops air-lifted into the South Pacific during World War II led to better understanding of body fluid regulation.

Intestinal losses are not "physiological" (as are losses from skin or lung), and are related to pathological states where vomiting or diarrhea occur.

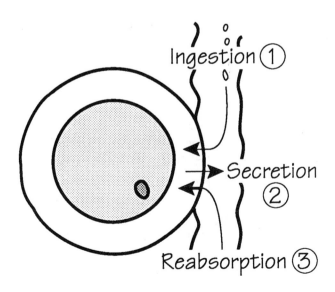

The normal intestine absorbs fluids that are ingested (1); secretes large amounts of digestive fluids (2); and then reabsorbs virtually all that it secretes (3).

The fluids in the intestine are separate from the E.C.F., but because of the large surface area of the intestinal mucosa and its close contact with the E.C.F. compartment, potential fluid losses from the E.C.F. into an abnormal intestine can be large.

If mucosal function is disturbed, the intestinal wall can cease to be a barrier to the E.C.F. with the result that diarrheal losses or losses into a dilated bowel, as in paralytic ileus, represent direct losses from the E.C.F.

3

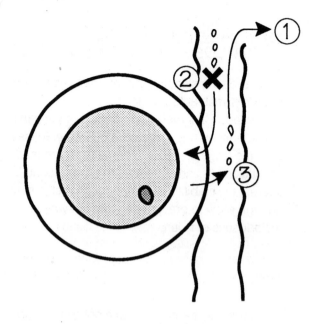

Vomiting:

Vomiting causes fluid loss in three ways:

1) By ejecting fluids already taken by mouth.

2) By limiting further intake of normal fluid volumes.

3) By the ejection of fluids secreted into the upper intestine, primarily the gastric juices.

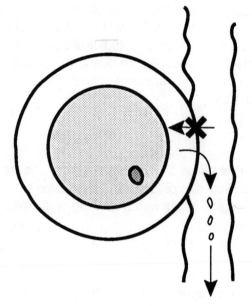

Diarrhea:

Diarrhea involves the failure to reabsorb the fluids secreted into the intestine and often a change in the permeability of the mucosa. This allows the intestine to become the site of what, in effect, are direct losses of E.C.F. The resultant intestinal losses (either up or down) tend to be isotonic with respect to the E.C.F.

It is only from the terminal part of the large intestine that diarrheal losses are hypotonic and therefore reflect losses of free water rather than E.C.F.

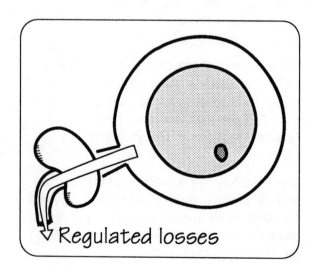

Regulated losses

The Kidney:

Losses from the lungs, skin and intestine are not open to tight physiologic control and are determined by changing environmental events.

Only the losses from the kidney can be regulated precisely and this organ therefore plays a crucial role in the regulation of the E.C.F. volume in health and disease.

Subdivision of E.C.F.

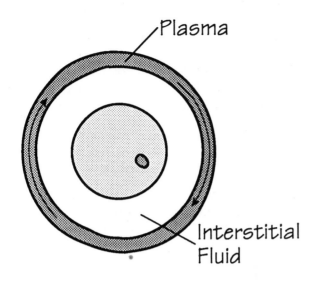

The E.C.F. is more complicated than we have indicated so far since it can be subdivided into two compartments.

One, the larger part, contains the interstitial fluid which surrounds the cells closely and intimately.

The second contains the plasma which, of course, circulates throughout the body and can therefore act as a "bulk transporter" of water and solutes in the E.C.F. It can also serve as a route for the even and rapid distribution of very small quantities of substances such as hormones and drugs. It is separated from the interstitial fluid by the walls of the capillaries.

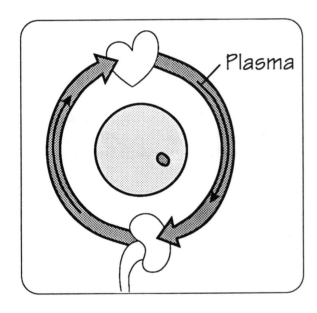

Circulation within the plasma compartment is uni-directional with the heart serving as the pump which ensures its continued movement.

In some diagrams we will show the plasma compartment as in this diagram which indicates the importance of the heart as a pump for the plasma and the kidney as a sensor and regulator of its volume.

The link between heart and kidney is precise and intimate. Mechanical factors (e.g. flow and pressure) neurogenic factors (via autonomic nerves) and humoral factors (e.g. aldosterone and atrial natriuretic peptide) provide this linkage.

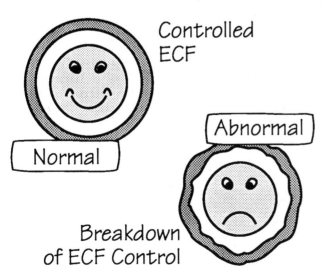

In normal health, changes in the volume and composition of the E.C.F. are within narrow limits and changes in the E.C.F. compartments complement each other.

In this setting, the I.C.F. is effectively protected from surrounding environmental change.

In abnormal clinical situations, changes in volume and composition of the E.C.F. become wider, and the balance between the E.C.F. compartments may become disturbed.

In this setting, the volume and composition of the E.C.F. varies outside narrow limits of tolerance and the cells can no longer rely upon a constant surrounding environment.

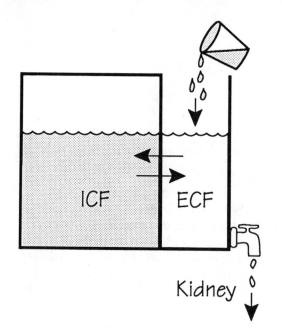

The Tank Model

Whilst in reality the E.C.F. surrounds the I.C.F. like a shell, it is often more convenient to depict the compartments as shown here.

The I.C.F. is drawn as a closed space which indicates that there are limits to its ability to expand, and that the only way into and out of the I.C.F. is via the E.C.F.

The tap represents the kidney and the horizontal wavy line the normal level of the fluid volume in each compartment.

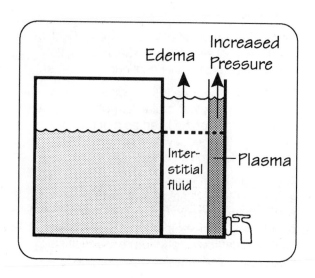

The E.C.F. includes the plasma and interstitial fluid compartments.

Expansion or contraction of these spaces can be recognized by such changes as the presence or absence of edema (for the interstitial space) or changes in venous or arterial pressure (the plasma space).

These will be reviewed in more detail in Chapter 3.

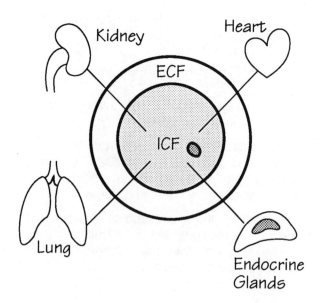

Cells as Regulators

Whilst the body cells in general are protected from environmental changes by the constancy of the E.C.F., some of the cells in the body are specially adapted to have a major role in regulating volume and composition of the E.C.F.

These include cells of organs such as the kidney, the lung, the heart and the endocrine glands.

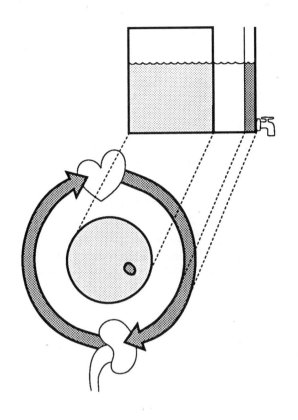

The Purpose of this Book

This book is about the body fluid compartments and the principles governing the regulation of both their volume and composition. It is concerned with concepts, and not with the details of distribution of every solute in every body compartment.

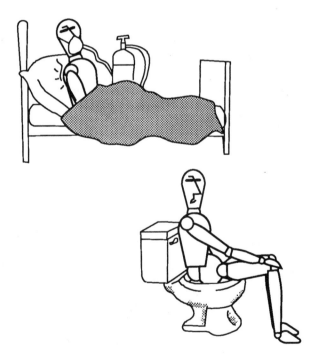

These concepts are fundamental to the understanding of the practical management of disorders of the body fluids. They can be related to such widely differing situations as heart failure and massive diarrhea due to cholera.

They can be applied to the understanding of diuretics, diabetes and drug distribution.

They are, quite simply, basic building blocks for good medicine.

Chapter 2

Coming to Terms with Terms

Before going any further into the distribution and regulation of fluids and electrolytes, it is important to understand their measurement and the units by which they are expressed. The problem here is that changes have occurred as the S.I. system of units has been introduced. "S.I." stands for Systeme International des Unités which attempts to relate all units of measurement to seven "base units". Where such units, together with the units derived from them, are applicable to clinical science they have been introduced as a rational advance. The rate at which these units have been introduced and accepted in clinical practice was more rapid in Europe than North America and the completeness with which they will be accepted is not yet clear. For these reasons, the terms used in clinical medicine are not "pure" and for the time being this is likely to remain the case. This chapter will attempt to clarify the concepts of current usage, with the understanding that the S.I. system is likely to become more widely used as time passes.

There remains a major dichotomy in North America where S.I. units are now universal in Canada but not in the United States. Those involved in clinical care must accept the need to be aware of both systems for some time to come.

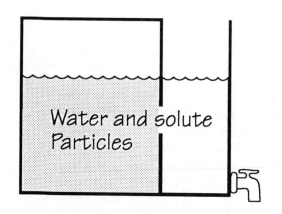

Body Fluids

All body fluids are aqueous solutions and therefore consist of water (the solvent) and dissolved particles (the solutes).

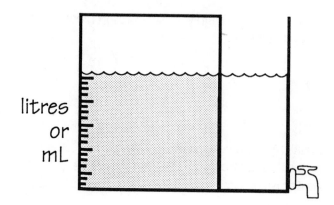

Water - The Solvent

When we talk about a "volume" we mean a volume of water and its dissolved solutes. Water can be regarded as the major solvent for biological systems. The volume occupying any "space" or "compartment" is measured in litres (L) or millimetres (mL).

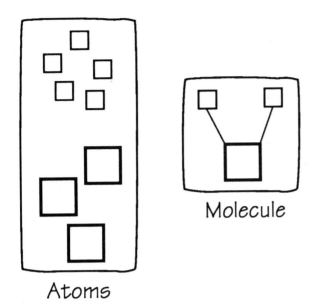

Atoms

Molecule

Solutes

The solutes in biological systems are minute particles which may be molecules or fragments of molecules.

Molecules

A **molecule** is the smallest particle into which a compound may be divided whilst still retaining its chemical identity.

Molecules are made up of collections of **atoms** which are electrically neutral with a balance between positive charges in the nucleus and negatively charged electrons in the outer shell.

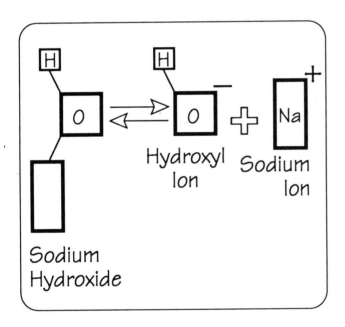

Hydroxyl Ion

Sodium Ion

Sodium Hydroxide

Ions

When molecules dissolve in water they may dissociate to a greater or lesser extent into their component parts which then carry electrical charges and are called **ions**. These ions may contain part of a single atom (such as sodium) or more than one atom (as in the hydroxyl ion).

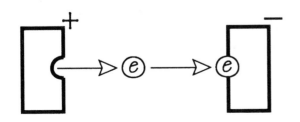

Positively charged ions have given up an electron, and negatively charged ions have gained an electron.

9

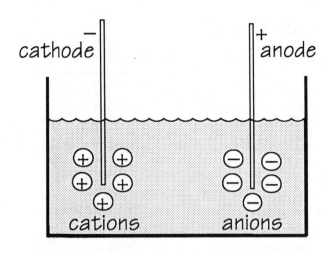

If electrodes are placed in a solution, the positively charged ions migrate to the cathode and are called **cations**. Negatively charged ions migrate to the anode and are called **anions**.

Cations are positively charged.

Anions are negatively charged.

Electrolytes

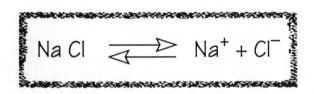

The interaction between the constituent ions of a substance in solution is an electrochemical one.

The charged nature of the particles in such a solution allows it to act as a conductor of electrical current. Such ionizing substances are therefore called **electrolytes**. Sodium chloride is an example of such a substance.

Valency

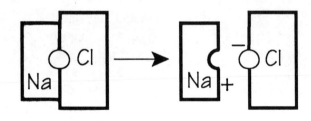

When sodium chloride dissociates, the chloride ion acquires one electron and becomes an anion, whilst the sodium ion loses one electron to become a cation.

Sodium and chloride are each **univalent** ions.

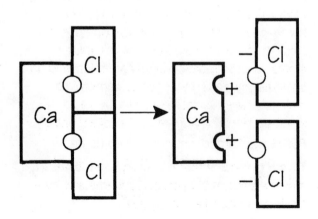

Calcium chloride, on the other hand, dissociates into one calcium ion with two positive charges and two chloride ions each with one negative charge.

Calcium is a **divalent** ion.

10

Hydrogen   Carbon

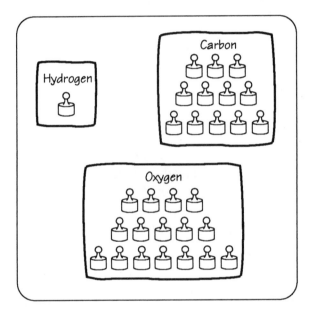

Atomic and Molecular Weights

The atoms which make up a substance can be related to one another in terms of mass (the **atomic weight**).

If the atomic weight of hydrogen is taken to be unity, then carbon has an atomic weight of 12, indicating that it is twelve times as heavy as hydrogen. Atomic weights are therefore masses relative to a reference atom and not actual weights.

Although the "reference atom" is, historically, hydrogen, carbon, with an atomic weight of 12, is now used as the absolute standard against which other atomic weights are compared.

Gram Atomic Weight

Atomic weights can be expressed in any unit of mass, but most commonly it is the gram. Thus, the gram atomic weight of hydrogen is 1 gram, and of carbon 12 grams, but since atomic weights are relative to one another any unit of mass can be used for comparison so long as the two atoms being compared are expressed in the same unit.

Whatever unit of mass is used, an atom of oxygen will always be sixteen times as heavy as hydrogen and one and a third times the mass of a carbon atom.

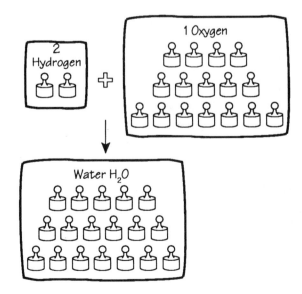

Gram Molecular Weight

Since molecules are made up of collections of atoms, their mass can be compared to one another as the **molecular weight**, which is the sum of the atomic weights of the constituent atoms. Just as atomic weights are relative to an absolute standard (hydrogen or carbon), so molecular weights are related to the same standard since they are made of collections of atoms.

Thus a molecule of water has eighteen times the mass of an atom of hydrogen and one and two-thirds the mass of a carbon atom.

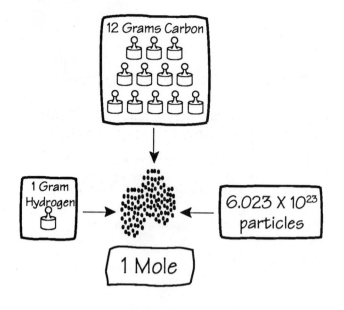

Mole - Amount of Substance

Measurements of the **amount** of any substance in biological systems is related to the basic composition of matter. The S.I. unit for amount is the **mole** (mol) which, not surprisingly, is related to the reference unit of atomic mass, namely carbon, (and thus indirectly to hydrogen).

A mole is the amount of any substance that contains the same number of particles as there are atoms in 12 grams of carbon. (For the purist, this number is 6.023×10^{23} particles and is referred to as Avagadro's number.)

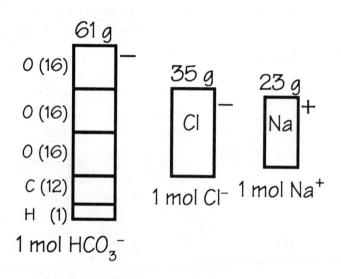

The particles may be atoms or molecules or ions, all of which can be measured in moles.

Thus, 61 grams of bicarbonate ions will contain the same number of particles as 35 grams of chloride ions, 23 grams of sodium ions and (of course) 12 grams of carbon atoms.

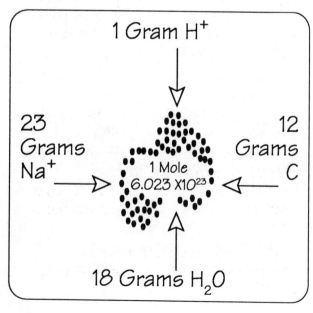

In practical terms, the gram molecular or atomic weight will contain the same number of particles as 12 grams of carbon. That is to say, the amount of substance in the gram molecular weight is one mole.

Similarly, the amount of substance in the gram atomic weight or the gram ionic weight is also one mole.

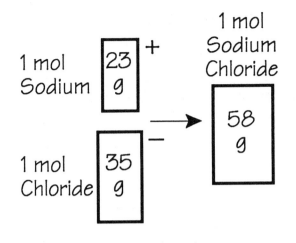

Sodium chloride can serve as an example.

The gram molecular weight is 58 grams. This is the sum of the gram atomic weight of sodium (23) and chloride (35).

Thus, 58 grams of sodium chloride contain one mole.

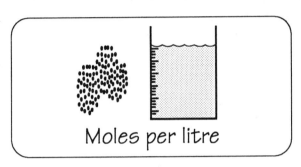

Moles per litre

When substances go into solution, their concentration is expressed as amount per volume and the units used are, of course, moles per litre (mol/L).

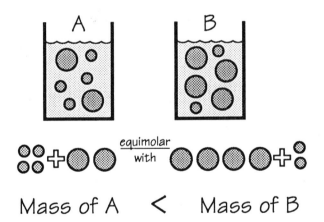

Mass of A < Mass of B

Because a mole is a number of particles rather than a mass of substance, solutions of equal molar concentration do not necessarily contain the same weight of solute.

The two solutions shown in this diagram are equimolar because they contain the same number of particles, but it is apparent that the heavier particles predominate in solution B and so the mass of solute in solution B is greater than the mass of solute in solution A.

mole (mol)

millimole (mmol) 10^{-3} mol
micromole (μmol) 10^{-6} mol
nanomole (nmol) 10^{-9} mol
picomole (pmol) 10^{-12} mol

In biological systems amounts of substances are often fractions of moles, and they are commonly expressed as thousandths (10^{-3}) of a mole (millimoles or mmol), 10^{-6} mole (micromoles or μmol), 10^{-9} mole (nanomoles or nmol), or occasionally 10^{-12} mole (picomoles or pmol).

In solution, their concentrations will be expressed as fractions of a mole per litre (e.g. mmol/L).

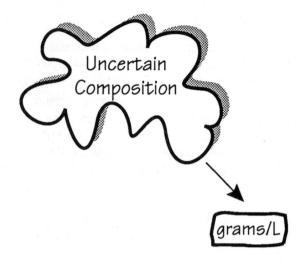

What has been said so far, although true of any substance, is only applicable to substances of known composition and therefore of known atomic or molecular weight.

One cannot use the term mole as a measure of amount of substance if one does not know the precise composition of the substance.

Many biological compounds have a complex and unknown chemical structure and for these substances, we will still have to use the term grams per litre for the expression of concentration. In fact, such compounds are more likely to be expressed as milligrams per decilitre.

Equivalents

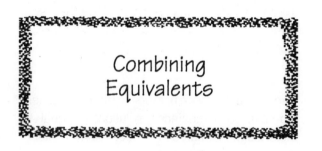

The concept of "combining equivalents" has been widely used in clinical practice. With the introduction of S.I. units, the term "equivalent" has been to a large extent replaced by mole (expressed as the gram ionic weight of a substance).

But the term "equivalent" is still of use because of its value in linking mass and charge in reactions between ions; although it is not an S.I. unit, it is so widely used and conceptually valuable that it is likely to continue in use for the time being.

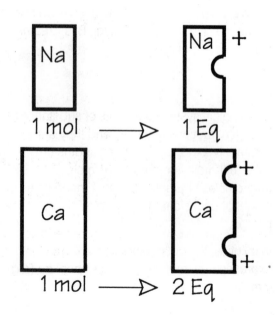

This concept relates the ionic weight of an electrolyte to the number of charges it carries (the valency).

The equivalent weight of an ion is the atomic mass divided by the valence. This means that for a univalent ion like sodium 1 mole contains 1 equivalent.

For a divalent ion such as calcium 1 mole contains 2 equivalents.

Since for univalent ions one millimole is the same as one milliequivalent (mEq), the terms mmol and mEq are interchangeable.

But for divalent ions milliequivalents and millimoles are **not** interchangeable. In most situations, confusion is avoided by using the term mole rather than equivalent.

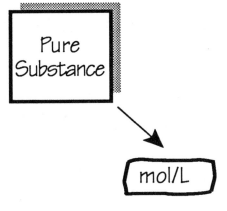

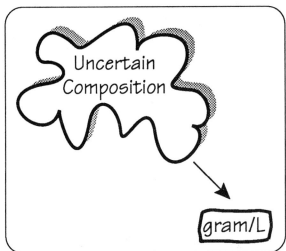

Plasma Conc.	Traditional	S.I.
Calcium	10mg/dl	2.5mmol/L
Magnesium	1.0mEq/L	0.5mmol/L
Sodium	140mEq/L	140mmol/L
Chloride	100mEq/L	100mmol/L

Plasma Conc.	Traditional	S.I.
Bilirubins	1mg/dl	18μmol/L
Urea	*10mg/dL	3.6mmol/L
Creatinine	1mg/dL	88μmol/L
Glucose	100mg/dL	5.5mmol/L

*expressed as Urea Nitrogen

S.I. Units - a Summary

In S.I. units, the concentrations of substances of known and exact composition are expressed as moles (or fractions of a mole) per litre.

Substances of ill defined composition, such as proteins, continue to be expressed by weight and their concentration as weight/L. So the terms gram/litre (g/L) and milligrams/litre (mg/L) will be used.

Terms such as "mg%" and "mg/100 ml" are more accurately stated as "mg/dL" (where "dL" is a decilitre).

This means that we have had to become accustomed to changes in the units for a number of substances, although those that we have traditionally expressed in molar terms will, of course, not alter.

Amongst the electrolytes, sodium and chloride have not changed.

Calcium and magnesium, which have often been expressed as mg/dl, or mEq/L, are expressed in molar terms (mmol/L).

Amounts of pure substances other than electrolytes have also been changed to molar terms and the ranges we have previously used clinically have changed very strikingly.

Thus, urea is now expressed in molar terms rather than the unsatisfactory traditional way of expressing it as "mg of nitrogen per decilitre".

A number of non-S.I. terms are likely to continue in use. We have already mentioned the continued use of equivalents as one of these. Another is the concept of pH as a way of expressing hydrogen ion activity rather than using molar concentrations of hydrogen ions. This will be discussed further at the end of this chapter.

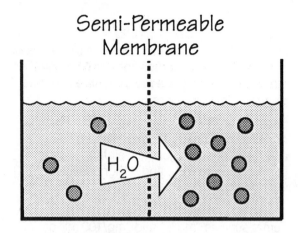

Semi-Permeable Membrane

Osmotic Activity

Osmosis refers to the movement of water (the solvent) across a membrane from a solution of lower concentration to a solution of higher concentration. The membrane concerned must be permeable to water but effectively impermeable to the solute.

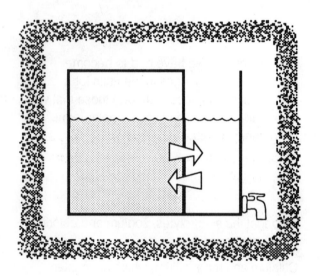

Water can move freely throughout the body compartments and its distribution is dependent upon osmotic forces which, if left to reach equilibrium, will result in the concentration of particles on each side of a membrane being equal. The distribution of particles (and thus of water) depends on the permeability of the membrane and the size of the particles concerned.

The tendency for water to move along concentration gradients can be measured in terms of the hydrostatic pressure required to prevent such movement. Thus, osmotic pressure can be measured in millimeters of mercury.

The number of particles in a solution determines the osmotic activity of that solution and can be expressed in terms of osmoles or milliosmoles and measured by determining the degree to which the freezing point of the solution is depressed.

Where osmotic effects (as opposed to chemical or electrical effects) are being considered, the units **osmole** (osmol) and **milliosmole** (mosmol) are used.

Non-Ionizing Substances

For a compound that does not dissociate, such as glucose or urea, the number of osmotically active particles will equal the number of molecules and therefore 1 millimole is equivalent to 1 milliosmole.

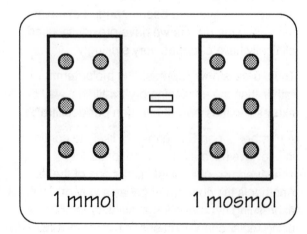

1 mmol = 1 mosmol

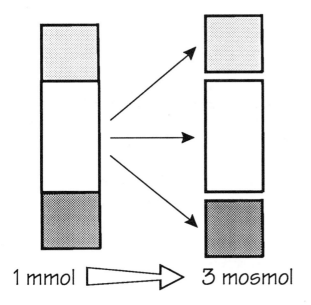

1 mmol ⟹ 3 mosmol

Ionizing Substances

In the case of a compound that does dissociate, one molecule will break up into more than one particle. Thus, in solution, 1 millimole will produce more than 1 milliosmole, in the case shown in this illustration 3 milliosmoles.

It is important to recognize that measurement of the number of particles in a solution (its osmolal concentration) tells nothing about its osmotic activity which only takes effect when the solution is exposed to an adjacent solution across a semi-permeable barrier.

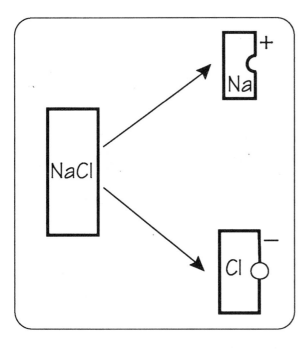

Thus for a substance like sodium chloride which breaks up into a positively charged sodium ion and a negatively charged chloride ion, 1 millimole would generate 2 milliosmoles in solution (provided complete dissociation occurred).

Osmotic Coefficient

In practice the dissociation of sodium chloride is often accepted as being complete. In fact it dissociates about 90% completely and has an osmotic coefficient of about 0.9. This value will vary to a small extent depending upon the concentration of the solution.

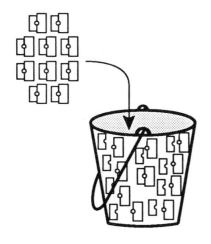

This means (using round figures for simplicity) that if we were to drop 10 molecules of sodium chloride into a beaker of water, they would break up into 19 particles: nine sodium ions, nine chloride ions and one sodium chloride molecule.

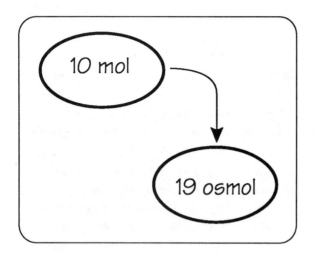

Thus 10 moles would yield 19 osmoles and 1 millimole would generate 1.9 milliosmoles. Preparing a solution of an ionizing solute with a pre-determined concentration of particles is not a simple matter of weighing out a given amount and dissolving it in water.

This will give a solution containing a pre-determined amount (mol/L) but the number of particles depends upon an osmotic coefficient which varies with the ionic concentration of the solution.

Osmolality or Osmolarity?

The concentration of particles in a solution can be expressed either as its osmolarity or as its osmolality.

An osmolar solution contains 1 osmole dissolved in water and made up to one litre of solution. Osmolarity thus refers to a concentration of active particles in a litre of solution.

An **osmolal** solution contains one osmole dissolved in a kilogram of water. Osmolality thus refers to a concentration of active particles in a kilogram of water.

For a pure solution of sodium chloride, for instance, the difference is so small that the two terms are effectively interchangeable.

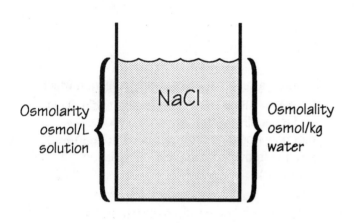

However, for a more complicated solution, such as plasma, the situation is less simple. Of a given volume of plasma, 10% is made up of solids (including proteins, lipids, urea and glucose) rather than water. As a result, osmolality and osmolarity are appreciably different: the osmolality is greater than the osmolarity because a litre of plasma only contains about nine tenths of a kilogram of water rather than a full kilogram.

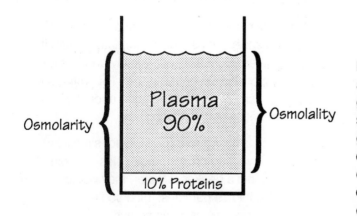

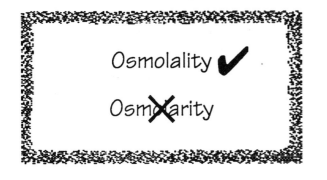

Since osmotic activity depends upon the concentration of active particles per kilogram of water, the term osmolality is the correct one to use and is the quantity measured by osmometers. Osmolarity is therefore a technically incorrect and inaccurate term.

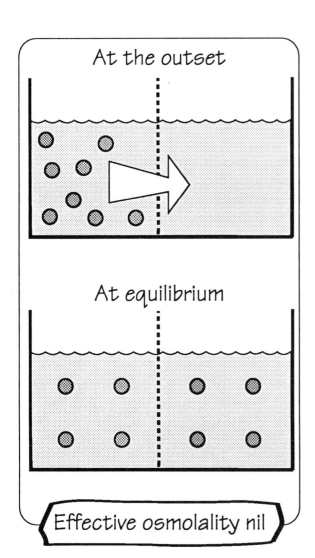

Effective Osmolality

If two compartments are separated by a membrane with water on either side and a solute is put into one compartment, it will only exert an osmotic effect if the particles stay on one side.

If they are small and very permeant, they will rapidly diffuse across the membrane and abolish any osmotic gradient. Thus the effective osmolality of such a solution rapidly becomes nil. The calculated osmolality of such a solution produces no long term effect because biological membranes are permeable to the solute.

Urea is such a solute. Only in very unusual clinical situations does urea exert any generalized osmotic effects and such effects are very transient.

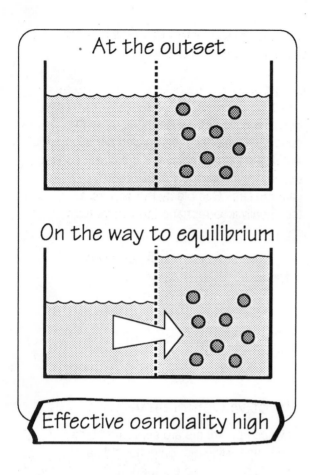

At the outset

On the way to equilibrium

Effective osmolality high

If, on the other hand, the solute particles are too large to pass through the membrane they will exert an osmotic effect. Colloids such as proteins are like this and they exert effective osmolality. A volume of water will move from one compartment to another to equalize the osmolality.

In man this principle is the major factor determining the balance of volume between the plasma and the interstitial fluid.

Effective osmolality depends on the size of the solute particle and the permeability of the membrane.

Gibbs-Donnan Equilibrium

A special effect may occur in situations where fluid in one compartment contains small diffusible ions together with large non-diffusible ions like protein, which is anionic and can be designated Pr⁻.

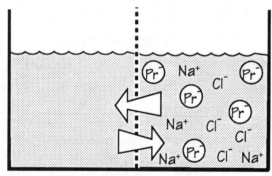

Without the presence of protein, electrochemical and osmotic forces would result in equal distribution of the small diffusible ions across the membrane.

But because the large protein ions cannot diffuse across, their presence causes an asymmetry of distribution of the small ions.

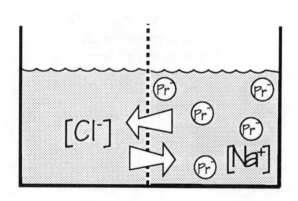

Anions, like chloride, will be in larger concentration on the side opposite to the protein, whilst cations, such as sodium, will be in higher concentration in the compartment containing protein.

Putting it another way, the negatively charged proteins attract the positively charged sodium and repel the negatively charged chloride.

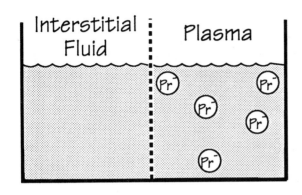

This kind of asymmetry is an example of the Gibbs-Donnan Equilibrium.

It explains in part the difference in effective osmotic pressure between the plasma and the interstitial fluid; since plasma albumin is a protein which cannot diffuse out of the capillaries, it thus produces an effective osmotic pressure partly due to its own small osmolar contribution and partly due to asymmetry of distribution of small diffusible ions that it produces.

This total osmotic effect of a non-diffusible colloid is called the **oncotic** pressure.

Tonicity

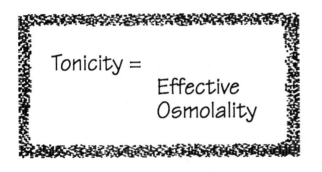

The term tonicity refers to the effective osmolality of a solution.

The two terms are interchangeable and relate to the osmotic effects when the solution is delivered to a biological setting. Thus, the measured osmolality of a bottle of sodium chloride solution becomes relevant only when it is infused into a patient.

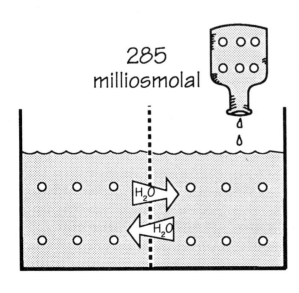

Isotonic Solutions

Isotonic solutions have the same effective osmolality as body fluids, that is they are close to 285 milliosmolal. Thus isotonic sodium chloride must also be close to 285 milliosmolal and this osmotic activity will be provided by a sodium chloride solution that is 154 millimolal.

This has been calculated as:

$$(154 \times 2)\,0.93$$

where 0.93 is the approximate osmotic coefficient for sodium chloride at this concentration.

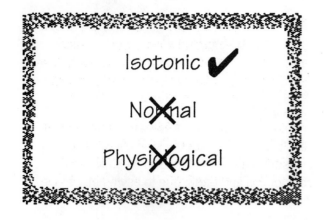

Isotonic sodium chloride is also known as "normal saline" and "physiological saline".

These two terms are of historic importance and are still often used. However, the more precise and functionally correct term is "isotonic sodium chloride".

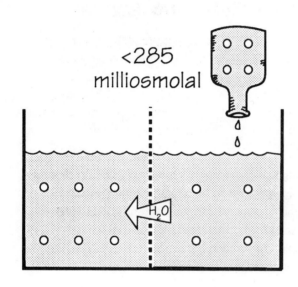

Hypotonic Solutions

Hypotonic fluids have a lower osmolality than body fluids. One solution, in clinical use, contains 77 millimoles of sodium chloride per litre and has exactly half the osmolality of isotonic sodium chloride. It is often referred to as "half normal saline".

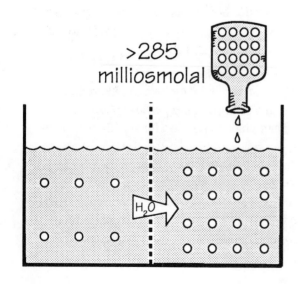

Hypertonic Solutions

Hypertonic solutions have an effective osmolality greater than that of body fluids. Such solutions may contain electrolytes (e.g. hypertonic sodium chloride) or non-electrolytes which have an osmotic effect because they do not diffuse across biological membranes (e.g. Mannitol).

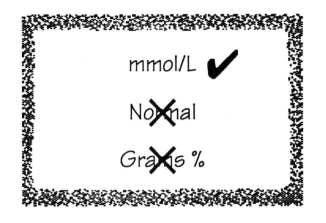

Clinicians often use terms such as "half normal saline" or "five percent saline" but it means much more in physiologic terms to refer to them as 77 mmol/L sodium chloride or 855 mmol/L sodium chloride respectively.

It is obvious that expressing all concentrations in terms of mmol/L is both consistent and eminently rational; it also avoids potentially dangerous confusion which, in clinical care, is an important consideration.

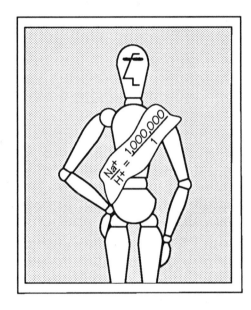

Hydrogen Ions and pH

Free hydrogen ions are present in most body fluids in very small concentrations. Blood plasma contains about 40 nanomoles of hydrogen ions per litre (i.e. 40×10^{-9} mol/L). This is roughly one millionth of the concentration of ions such as sodium and chloride.

Most hydrogen ions are bound to buffers, many of them within the cells and thus whilst there are relatively large amounts of hydrogen ions in the body, only a very few are freely circulating at any one time.

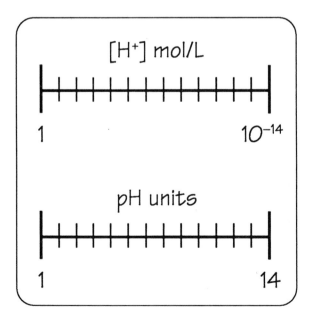

The concept of "pH" was developed by Sorenson to express free hydrogen ion concentration more compactly. Hydrogen ion concentration might range from 1 molar to 10^{-14} molar, an enormously wide range, far too wide for most clinical applications.

pH is defined by the following equation:

$$pH = \log \frac{1}{[H^+]}$$

It is a measure of hydrogen ion activity in a solution; usually it is measured by a hydrogen ion sensitive glass electrode and a "pH meter". A range of hydrogen ion concentration from one molar to 10^{-14} molar is thus described more simply by a range of pH from 1 to 14.

Fluid	pH*	[H+]
0.1 molar HCl	1	10^{-1} mol
Water	7.0	10^{-7} mol
Plasma	7.4	4×10^{-8} mol
0.1 molar NaOH	13	10^{-13} mol

*at 20° C

The concept of pH has been useful since it expresses such a wide range of hydrogen ion concentrations so conveniently; it also expresses hydrogen ion activity rather than merely the concentration of hydrogen ions.

Whether or not pH eventually becomes replaced by hydrogen ion concentration as S.I. units are implemented, pH is still likely to continue as a valued concept.

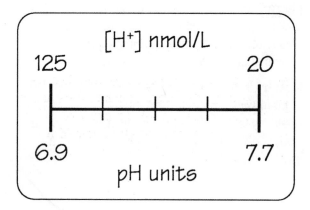

In clinical situations, hydrogen ion concentrations can vary from 125 to 20 nanomoles per litre. This represents a pH range from 6.9 to 7.7 but at each extreme life comes under grave threat.

This range, therefore, is much wider than the normally tolerated physiologic variations.

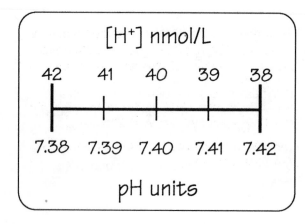

The physiologic range lies between a pH of 7.38 and 7.42 (a hydrogen ion concentration between 42 and 38 nanomoles per litre).

Within this range each change of 0.01 pH unit is equivalent to a change of hydrogen ion concentration of 1 nanomole per litre.

Chapter 3

The Distribution of Body Fluids

This chapter outlines the way in which water is distributed throughout the body, and explores some of the basic rules governing its transfer from one compartment to another.

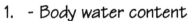

> 1. - Body water content
> 2. - Distribution between E.C.F. and I.C.F.
> 3. - Distribution of Solutes - electrochemical and osmotic activity
> 4. - Distribution between plasma and interstitial fluid

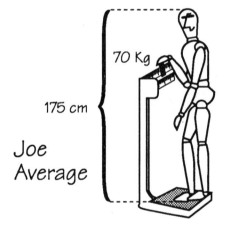

70 Kg

175 cm

Joe Average

Body Water Content

When we talk about "the average man", we are talking by convention about a male who is about 175 centimetres tall and weighs about 70 kilograms. Such a man contains about 60% water by weight.

In many clinical situations, you will not be dealing with "average" people; they may be fatter or thinner, and this will influence the size of their fluid compartments.

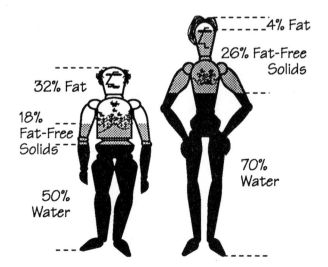

4% Fat

26% Fat-Free Solids

32% Fat

18% Fat-Free Solids

50% Water

70% Water

With one exception, all body tissues contain far more water than anything else. The exception is adipose tissue which contains only about 20% water.

Thus, obesity has a significant impact upon the amount of water an individual contains.

A fat man contains proportionately less water than does a thin man.

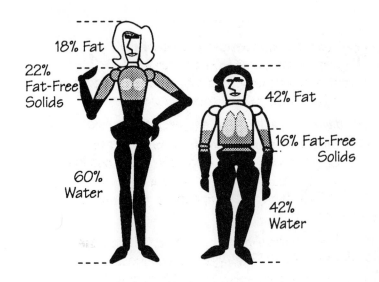

18% Fat
22% Fat-Free Solids
60% Water

42% Fat
16% Fat-Free Solids
42% Water

There is a gender difference, too, because women have proportionately more body fat than men. This means, by and large, women contain less water in proportion to their body weight than do men.

There are also, of course, differences between fat and thin women.

These are not usually major considerations in clinical medicine, but there are circumstances where these variations can be very significant.

Total Body Water*

	Infant	Male	Female
Thin	80	65	55
Average	70	60	50
Fat	65	55	45

*as % of body weight

This table shows how big the variation can be between infants, and adult males and females.

An infant may have as much as 80% of its body weight as water, and a malnourished infant who is depleted of fat may have even more than that.

This becomes very important because a child is much more vulnerable to the effects of volume depletion than an adult and what may be a trivial fluid loss for a normal adult may be a catastrophic loss, in percentage terms, for a child.

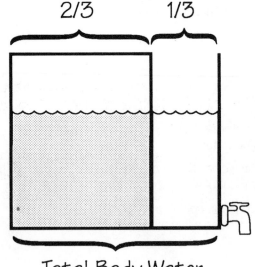

2/3   1/3

Total Body Water

Distribution of Water Between E.C.F. and I.C.F.

As described in chapter one, the body fluids can be divided into an intracellular compartment (I.C.F.) and an extracellular compartment (E.C.F.).

Approximately two thirds of body water will be inside the cells and one third outside the cells.

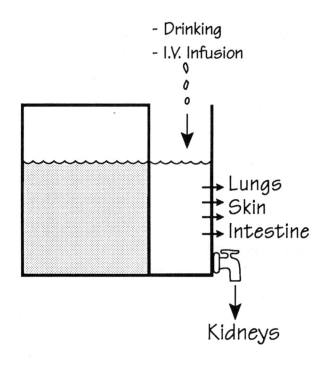

- Drinking
- I.V. Infusion

Lungs
Skin
Intestine

Kidneys

Normally, additions to the extracellular compartment are made by drinking, but physicians often add to it by unphysiologic routes, such as intravenous infusion.

Fluid can be lost from the extracellular compartment via a number of routes; these include losses via the lungs, the sweat, and the intestine, but the route of loss that is physiologically most important is from the kidney.

All such losses occur from the E.C.F., and the intracellular compartment can only lose or gain volume via the extracellular compartment.

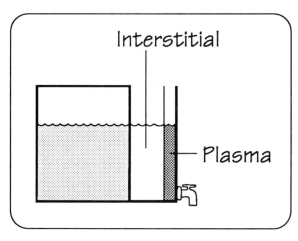

Interstitial

Plasma

About a quarter of the total E.C.F. is confined to the vascular space where it comprises the plasma volume.

The remaining three quarters is in the interstitial space outside the blood vessels and bathing the tissues.

These proportions are what you expect in an "average" adult and will vary with age, gender and fatness.

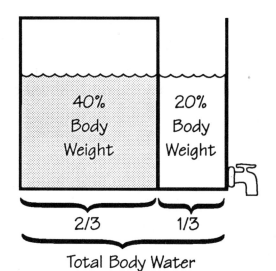

40% Body Weight

20% Body Weight

2/3   1/3

Total Body Water

The diagrams used here have shown that two thirds of total body water is in the I.C.F. and one third in the E.C.F.

In terms of total body weight this means that for a normal adult I.C.F. water constitutes 40% of body weight and E.C.F. water makes up 20% of body weight.

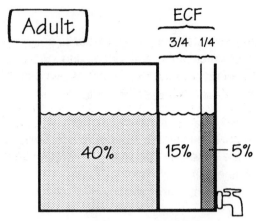

Total Body Water : 60% Body Wt.

In the adult the E.C.F. is divided so that three quarters of the fluid volume is interstitial and one quarter is in the plasma.

This means that interstitial water makes up 15% of body weight and plasma water 5% of body weight.

Small amounts of water are bound in dense fibrous tissue (e.g. tendons) and bone matrix. This water is not readily mobilized and is a small proportion of total body water. To avoid unnecessary complications it will not be considered further here.

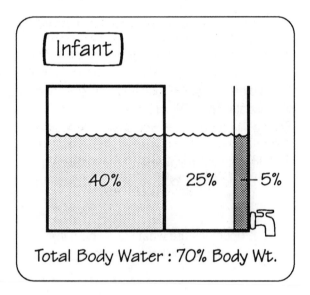

Total Body Water : 70% Body Wt.

In an infant, however, there is much more water (about 70% by weight). The proportion of water within the cells and within the plasma volume is exactly the same as in an adult, but the big difference is that an infant has a relatively larger interstitial volume. The ratio between interstitial and plasma volume is about 5:1 compared with 3:1 in the adult.

For an infant weighing only 5 kilograms and with a total body water of 3.5 litres a loss of one litre from the intestine (a small volume for an adult) may represent virtually the total E.C.F. volume.

Measuring the Volume of Compartments

Given a compartmental system of this kind, it is theoretically possible to measure the volume of any given compartment.

Such a measurement requires a marker which

1) Can be measured accurately
2) Is confined to the compartment whose volume is to be measured

The volume of the compartment containing the marker can then be measured by the degree to which the marker is diluted.

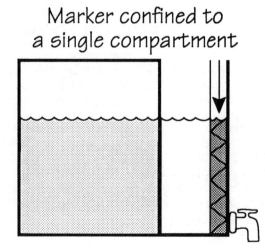

Marker confined to a single compartment

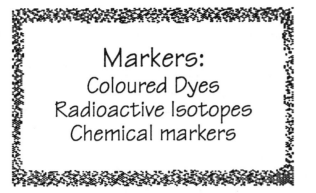

Markers:
Coloured Dyes
Radioactive Isotopes
Chemical markers

Markers may be radioactive isotopes such as ^{125}I-albumin which is (initially at least) distributed in the plasma volume. They may be chemical markers, such as thiocyanate, which is distributed throughout the E.C.F. No marker is absolutely confined to a single compartment, but suitably selected markers can provide reasonably close approximations which are of practical use.

Distribution of Solutes

In looking at the composition of the fluids within the body compartments we are interested predominantly in substances present in large amounts which have a major impact on either the electro-chemical or the osmotic activity within each compartment.

In all body fluids, whatever, their composition, anions and cations will always be present in equal amounts since positive and negative charges must be equal. This is a non-negotiable electrochemical reality.

A Biological Rule

Negative Charges = Positive Charges

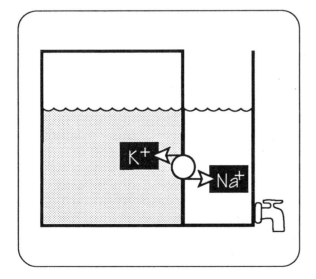

Cations

Sodium is the predominant cation in the extracellular space whilst in the intracellular space potassium is the predominant cation.

In complex animals like man, the cell wall has a pump system which pushes out the sodium that tends to leak in and pumps in the potassium that tends to leak out.

As long as the extracellular fluid compartment is maintained at a constant composition, the cells can also maintain a constant composition by mechanisms which utilize the energy provided by cellular metabolism and the mediation of membrane bound ATP-ase.

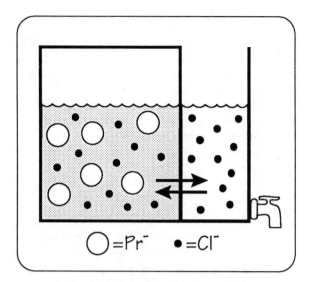

$\bigcirc = Pr^-$ $\bullet = Cl^-$

Anions

Within the cells the important anions are large organic molecules such as proteins together with phosphates. Proteins remain within the cell and are too large to diffuse out.

The main extracellular anions are chloride and bicarbonate.

Chloride is not exclusively outside the cells and distributes according to electrical forces. Since many of the cellular anions cannot diffuse out, chloride tends to end up predominantly outside the cells.

The Donnan Effect:

The asymmetry of distribution of a diffusible ion (chloride) due to the presence within the cell of a non-diffusible ion (protein) is another example of the Donnan effect (see page 20).

Distribution of Ions determines:

1. Electrical activity on cell surface
2. Osmotic pressure in compartments

The presence of small, charged, ionic particles in body fluids is vital to the function of the body, determining factors such as the surface charges on the cell walls (largely due to a leak of potassium from the cell), and the osmotic activity of each compartment.

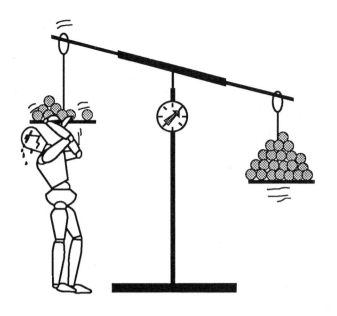

Osmolality of Body Fluids

As a general rule, osmotic gradients are not allowed to persist in the body, and water will move from one space to another along gradients determined by the distribution of solute ions.

Only in very special situations are osmotic gradients maintained to solve physiologic problems. Such a situation exists in the renal tubule where osmotic gradients are used to allow the recovery of free water from the glomerular filtrate (see chapter 7).

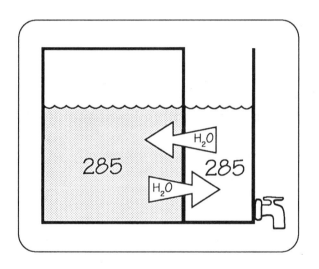

In man, therefore, the intracellular and extracellular fluids are of comparable osmolality and normally this is about 285 milliosmoles per kilogram.

Water, therefore, will move equally in either direction across the cell wall since the random movement of water molecules will be the same in each direction.

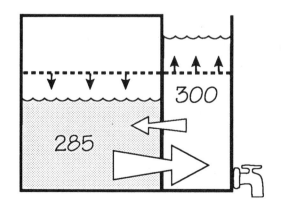

But suppose that the osmolality of the E.C.F. should become 300. There is now an osmotic gradient, and water moves predominantly from the cells into the E.C.F. until there is equalization of the osmotic pressure.

Thus osmotic factors exert control over the distribution of volume between compartments.

31

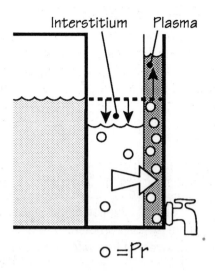

$\circ = Pr$

Distribution of Volume in the E.C.F.

The plasma and interstitial components of the E.C.F. are separated by the capillary walls which are freely permeable to both water and solutes, but only slightly permeable to proteins.

The distribution of sodium, chloride and other ions through the whole of the E.C.F. would be expected to be uniform, but because within the capillaries there is a higher concentration of protein, there is a relative osmotic gradient between the interstitium and the plasma; water and solutes tend to move constantly from the interstitial space into the plasma space in an attempt to balance the oncotic effect of the plasma proteins.

Unopposed, this effect would lead to an expanding plasma volume and a shrinking interstitial volume.

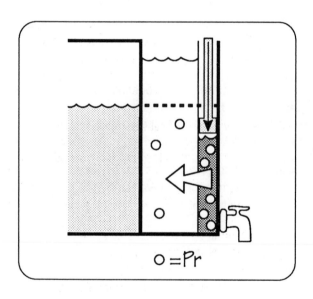

$\circ = Pr$

But another thing happens in the capillaries, especially at the arterial end.

Here there is a positive hydrostatic pressure inside the vessels which tends to push water and solutes, but not protein, into the interstitial space, tending to increase its volume at the expense of the plasma volume.

Unopposed, this effect would lead to an expanding interstitial volume and a shrinking plasma volume.

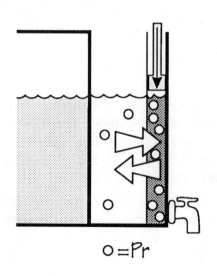

$\circ = Pr$

In normal circumstances, these two processes balance out and a steady state develops.

Osmotic factors tend to move fluid from the interstitial space into the plasma volume, and hydrostatic pressure tends to move it in the opposite direction.

The balance between these forces varies as the plasma flows along the smallest capillary blood vessels from arteriole to venule.

This concept was first enunciated by Starling in 1896.

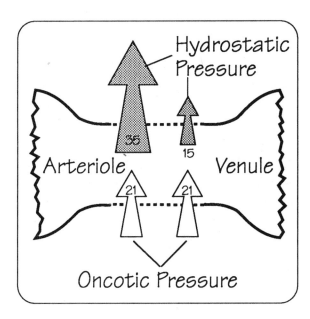

The Starling Hypothesis

At the arterial end of the capillary, fluids are filtered through its wall by hydrostatic pressures. Proteins (such as albumin) remain behind and exert an oncotic pressure which draws fluid back into the plasma. The balance favours movement from the plasma into the interstitium.

At the venous end of the capillary the hydrostatic pressure has fallen and the balance between hydrostatic and oncotic pressures now favours the return of fluids to the plasma from the interstitial space.

The result of these processes is a continuous movement of fluid across the capillary wall and the setting up of a balance between flow into and out of the plasma.

All pressures in this diagram are expressed as millimetres of mercury and are representative of an "average" capillary in the systemic circulation.

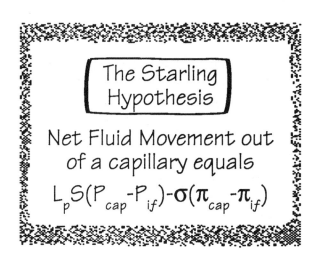

The Starling Hypothesis

Net Fluid Movement out of a capillary equals

$$L_p S(P_{cap} - P_{if}) - \sigma(\pi_{cap} - \pi_{if})$$

This concept can be expressed more completely by an equation which is shown opposite and includes the following terms.

- L_p — capillary permeability
- S — capillary surface area
- P_{cap} — capillary hydrostatic pressure
- P_{if} — interstitial hydrostatic pressure
- π_{cap} — plasma oncotic pressure
- π_{if} — interstitial oncotic pressure
- σ — the "reflection coefficient" of albumin across the capillary wall (unity means complete impermeability - zero means complete permeability).

Edema

The most striking clinical sign of a disordered balance of these forces in the capillary is the accumulation of water and solutes in the interstitial compartment, producing visible swelling (edema).

Firm pressure on such a swollen area will leave an impression - hence the clinical sign of "pitting" edema.

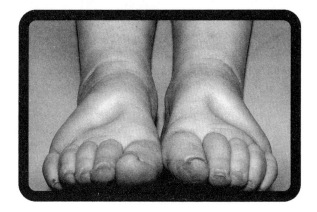

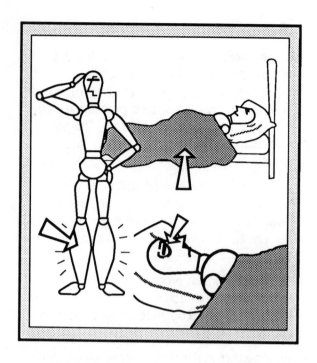

In states of generalized edema, the swelling is in the most dependent part; it is in the feet after a period of standing or walking, but of course it will end up in the face after some time lying flat. This is simply due to the effects of gravity added to the hydrostatic pressure in the capillaries.

This explains why many people with edema tend to have puffy eyes in the morning and puffy feet in the evening.

Patients lying in bed will accumulate edema over the sacrum and this may be missed by careless examination.

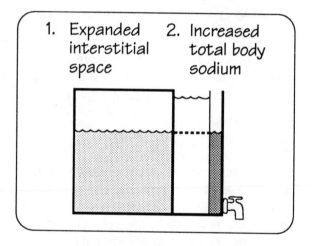

1. Expanded interstitial space   2. Increased total body sodium

One of the most important rules about edema, is that anybody who has generalized edema must have an expanded interstitial volume.

Since this volume is made up of water and the solutes present in the interstitial space, anyone who has edema of a generalized kind also has an increased total body sodium because sodium (and accompanying anions) are the major osmotically active E.C.F. solutes.

Edema and the Starling Concept

The beauty of the concepts involved in the distribution of fluid throughout the body is that they can be directly linked to a clinical setting. Thus, in thinking of the balance involved in the Starling hypothesis, it becomes obvious that edema can be caused by one (or more) of the following mechanisms:

1) An increased hydrostatic pressure in the capillaries. Examples of such a mechanism include venous occlusion (causing localized edema) and heart failure (causing generalized edema).

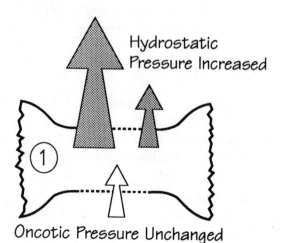

Hydrostatic Pressure Increased

Oncotic Pressure Unchanged

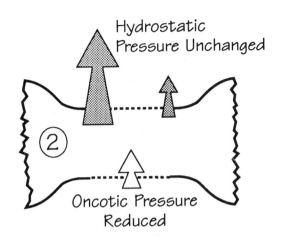

Hydrostatic
Pressure Unchanged

②

Oncotic Pressure
Reduced

2) A decrease in plasma oncotic pressure due to a reduction in its albumin concentration. Examples include protein loss from the kidney (nephrotic syndrome) or failure of hepatic synthesis of albumin. Such changes will always produce **generalized** edema.

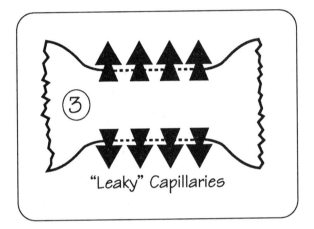

③

"Leaky" Capillaries

3) An increase in permeability of capillary walls will favour the production of edema. This usually occurs on a **localized** basis and explains the occurrence of edema at the site of an acute inflammatory reaction, for example, an insect bite or a cutaneous boil.

Edema and the Lymphatics

The Starling concept assumes that albumin remains within the plasma compartment.

Whilst, this is a realistic approximation, it is not an absolute fact. Albumin does, to some extent, leak out of the capillaries particularly when their permeability is altered by disease.

This problem is handled by the ubiquitous presence of lymphatic vessels running parallel to the capillary blood vessels. They are capable of taking up stray protein molecules and interstitial fluid and returning them to the plasma compartment via the central lymphatics and the thoracic duct.

When lymphatics are obstructed, edema will occur and will be distributed distal to the point of obstruction. Because of the increased protein content of the interstitial fluid in this situation "lymphatic edema" is firm and relatively non-pitting.

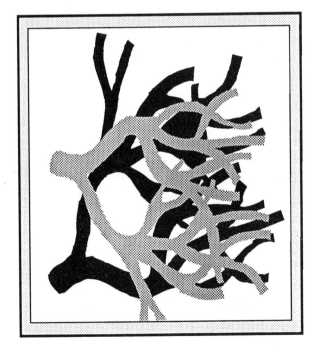

Chapter 4

The Regulation of Body Fluids

The regulation of fluid distribution within the body involves a series of co-ordinated responses to change, which all tend to maintain the constancy of volume and composition of the E.C.F. The more constant the environment provided by the E.C.F., the more will the cells be protected from changes in the external world.

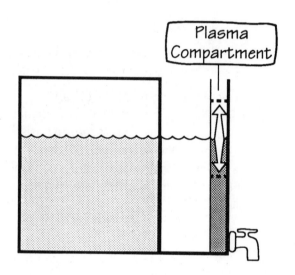

Changes in Plasma Volume

The plasma compartment has a relatively small volume, but the pressures and flows within it may be high. Shifts of volume and pressure within it may be rapid, for example in response to the gravitational effects caused by the simple expedient of rising from a lying to a standing position.

Direct loss of volume, such as occurs with hemorrhage will also be rapid especially from the arterial side where pressure and flow are highest.

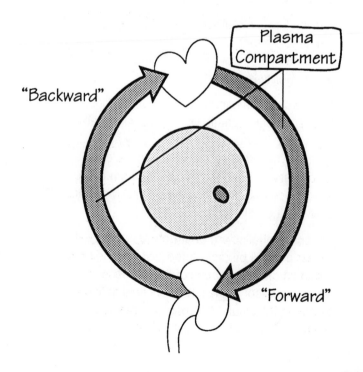

At this point it is important to modify the diagram of the plasma compartment that was developed in previous chapters. The circulation is, in mechanical terms, a closed system with uni-directional flow produced by the pumping heart.

Fluid (blood) is pumped continuously from the veins, behind the heart, to the arteries, in front of the heart.

This diagram shows the "forward" and "backward" parts of the plasma compartment as being equal.

This equality applies to rate of flow since cardiac output and input must be the same over a fixed time; however, it does not apply to volume and pressure which are markedly different.

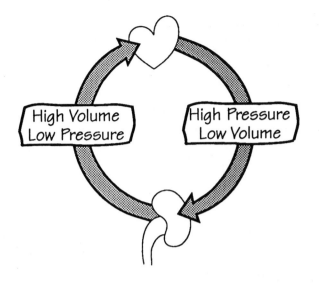

High Volume Low Pressure

High Pressure Low Volume

In fact, the "forward" circulation is a high pressure, low volume system, whilst the "backward" circulation is a high volume, low pressure system.

The smaller vessels "in front of" the heart (small arteries and arterioles) provide a resistance to blood flow and are called resistance vessels. Changes in their calibre in response to nervous and humoral stimuli cause changes in peripheral resistance which influence pressure and flow.

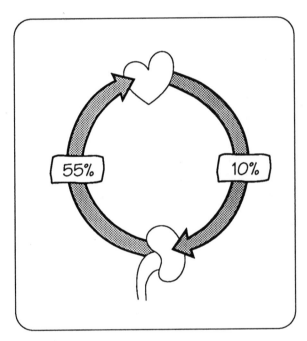

55%

10%

In the normal situation about 55% of the plasma volume is in the venous system whilst 10% is in the arterial system at any particular time. The remaining 35% is distributed in the heart, the lungs, and the capillary bed.

The large capacity of the venous system "behind" the heart allows it to accommodate an expanded volume with relatively much less change of pressure and flow than in the arterial system. For this reason veins are sometimes called capacitance vessels.

Clinically the volume of the "forward" part of the circulation can be assessed in terms of the pulse rate, blood pressure and temperature of the extremities.

Clinically the volume of the "backward" half can be assessed by the degree of filling of the jugular veins and the presence or absence of generalized edema.

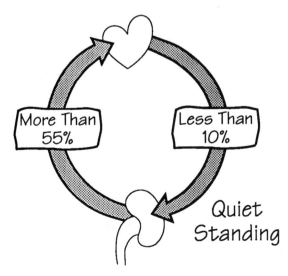

More Than 55%

Less Than 10%

Quiet Standing

Prolonged, quiet standing can produce increased venous pooling (due to gravitational forces) with a resultant reduction of the volume available to the arterial side of the circulation and thus a diminished blood flow to the key organs.

This is what happens to the soldier who faints on the parade ground. It is an example of the relatively rapid short-term change that can alter volume and flow in the plasma compartment and alter the distribution of blood between resistance and capacitance vessels.

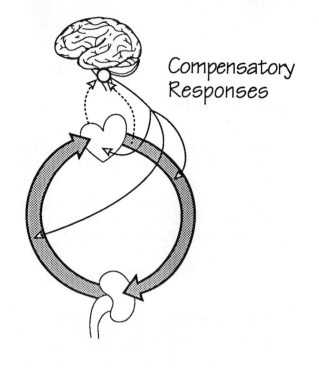

Compensatory Responses

These rapid and short-term changes in volume and flow are matched by equally rapid and short-term compensatory responses which minimize the effects of volume reduction or maldistribution.

These responses result from afferent information reaching the brain via nerve fibres from sensors in the heart and large blood vessels, such as the aortic stretch receptors.

This information is transmitted by efferent fibres in the autonomic nerves back to the heart and blood vessels which compensate by changes of cardiac output, arterial resistance and venous capacitance.

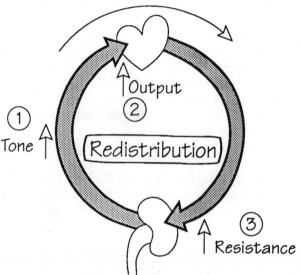

Thus, in the example of reduced venous return to the heart, and in response to altered afferent information, efferent stimuli will lead to changes that include:

1) increased venous tone,
2) increased cardiac output, and
3) increased arteriolar resistance.

All of these tend to allow blood to be redistributed from veins to arteries. These changes all result from the direct effects of autonomic nerve stimulation. They effectively correct the short-term changes in volume and flow that set them in motion in the first place.

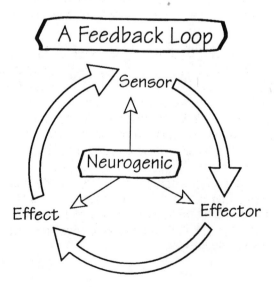

This is an example of a "feedback loop" which involves sensors which recognize change and effectors which correct it.

Such a feedback loop is a common concept in physiologic regulation and allows a continuous linkage between the output of a sensor and the effect which it produces.

In the case of the plasma volume, the initial responses to change are brisk and involve the rapid response of the autonomic nervous system.

38

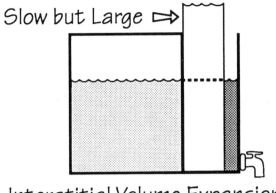

Slow but Large ⇒

Interstitial Volume Expansion

Changes in Interstitial Volume

Changes in interstitial volume may be, by contrast, much slower than changes of plasma volume; however, they may eventually be much larger.

The interstitial space may expand by many litres over a long period of time without producing any major functional disturbance within the plasma compartment or the I.C.F.

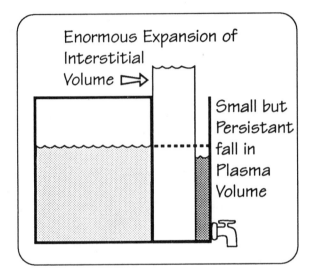

Enormous Expansion of Interstitial Volume ⇒

Small but Persistant fall in Plasma Volume

Such a change of interstitial volume occurs when a reduction of plasma albumin leads to a fall of oncotic pressure in the plasma with a consequent "shift" of volume into the interstitial compartment.

This results in a small but persistent fall in plasma volume which activates a series of regulating systems that result in retention of salt and water by the kidney. So long as the plasma albumin remains low, however, volume will continue to shift out of the plasma compartment and produce ever-increasing interstitial expansion. The persisting small change in plasma volume may produce no apparent effects of itself but the interstitial edema which results may be overwhelming.

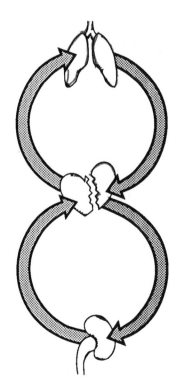

The balance between the plasma and interstitial compartments is more delicate in the pulmonary circulation. Our single circuit model is an over-simplification, and it can be redrawn to include a systemic and a pulmonary component of plasma volume.

The pulmonary circulation accommodates the same cardiac output as the systemic circulation but is more distensible and has a lower capillary hydrostatic pressure (about 10 mm Hg.). In addition, there is periodic subatmospheric pressure in the chest cavity, associated with breathing, which will be transmitted to the distensible blood vessels in the chest. Increases in pulmonary interstitial volume result in breathlessness and extravasation of fluid into the alveoli (pulmonary edema) which may be an early sign of E.C.F. volume expansion in some clinical situations.

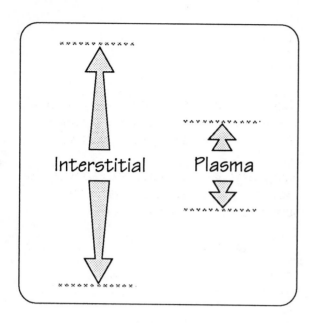

In summary:

1) The plasma cannot change very much in volume without inducing fairly striking compensatory vascular responses.

2) By contrast, the interstitial volume can expand (or contract) to a much greater degree, and if it does so slowly there may be relatively little functional disturbance until quite large changes have occurred.

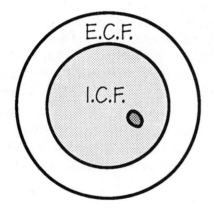

The important concept is that the E.C.F., as a whole, may vary within predetermined limits as the body reacts to its environment, but the I.C.F. remains extremely stable.

The E.C.F. interfaces with the outside world and becomes modified by it; the degree to which its composition is regulated by such organs as kidneys and lungs determines the degree to which the E.C.F. provides an optimum "bath" for the cells.

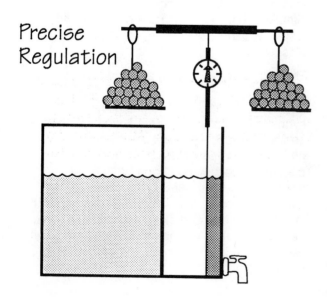

Precise Regulation

The Regulation of E.C.F. volume and osmolality

The body is equipped with mechanisms which allow the precise regulation of E.C.F. composition.

The most important concern regulation of the volume of water and the amount of sodium. These two components of the E.C.F. determine its volume and its osmolality and in turn determine the movement of water in and out of the cells.

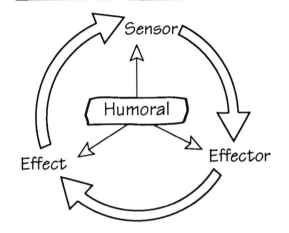

Another Feedback Loop

Sensor, Humoral, Effect, Effector

Two of the best understood of these regulatory mechanisms will be introduced here and described in more detail in later chapters.

Both of them involve a feedback loop but in this case the effectors are circulating humoral agents rather than autonomic nerves.

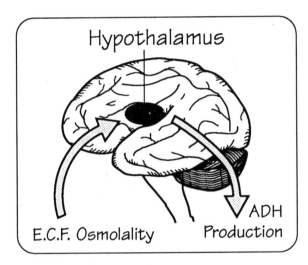

Hypothalamus

E.C.F. Osmolality → ADH Production

1. Osmotic Regulation- Water and Antidiuretic Hormone

One sensor is a group of specialized cells in the hypothalamus which recognize changes of osmolality in the surrounding E.C.F. As a result, they regulate the amount of the peptide anti-diuretic hormone (ADH) released from the hypothalamus. Minor changes in osmolality (which are constantly occurring) lead to minor changes in ADH production.

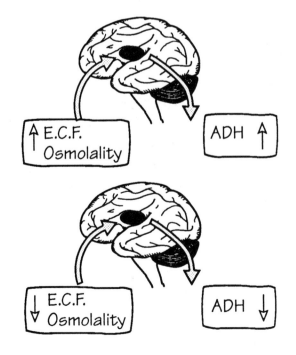

↑ E.C.F. Osmolality → ADH ↑

↓ E.C.F. Osmolality → ADH ↓

A rising osmolality increases ADH production, a falling osmolality reduces it. In normal living, with intermittent salt and water intake, these two components (osmolality and ADH production) are in constant interaction, both moving within limits which we call "physiological".

41

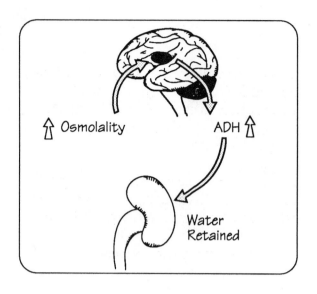

ADH promotes the retention of water by the kidney. As a result, the urine volume falls and its concentration rises. As ADH secretion rises, so water retention by the kidney increases.

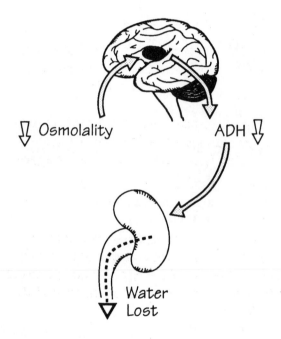

Conversely, the less ADH that is secreted, the more water is lost, the urine volume rises and its concentration falls. Thus, varying ADH release results in a variation of water loss that precisely matches the variations of osmolality in the E.C.F.

Thus the "feedback loop" is closed. Osmolality is kept within tight limits by the interaction of a hypothalamic sensor and a renal effector, with ADH acting as an intermediary.

The details of this mechanism will be discussed in Chapter 7.

2. Volume Regulation- Aldosterone

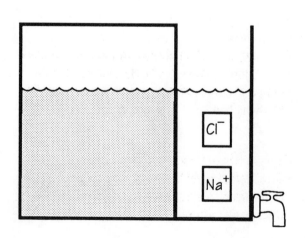

Other sensors are concerned with changes in volume rather than changes in osmolality. In this regard, it is important to remind the reader that sodium and its accompanying anions (predominantly chloride) are effectively confined to the E.C.F. By their osmotic effect within the E.C.F. they determine the volume of that compartment. Thus, the amount of sodium in the E.C.F. determines the volume of the E.C.F.

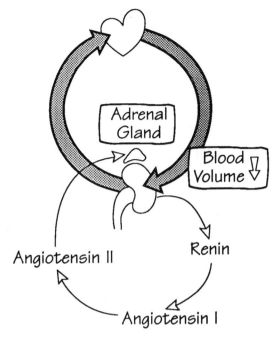

The systems concerned with regulating volume, are concerned with the regulation of E.C.F. sodium content and one of the most important ones activates the "renin-angiotensin-aldosterone system."

This involves a series of steps in a cascade that begins with diminution of blood volume or flow being sensed by specialized cells within the kidney and results in the secretion of aldosterone from the adrenal gland.

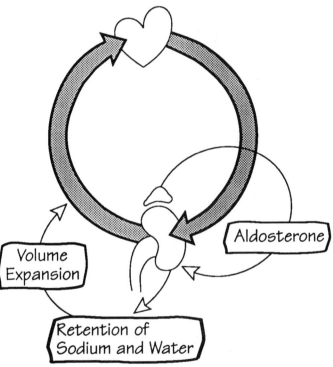

The feedback loop is completed as aldosterone causes the kidney to retain sodium (and with it water) to correct the volume deficit.

The reverse process results in the loss of salt and water by the kidney in states of volume expansion. Details of this mechanism are given on pages 70-72.

These concepts will be developed further in chapters 6 and 7. They have been simplified here for the sake of clarity, but in fact are linked together in complex ways that are not yet fully understood.

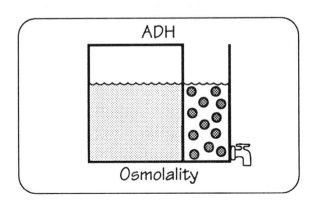

For example, ADH secretion can be stimulated by "volume" stimuli, probably arising from the heart and great vessels, as well as by osmotic stimuli.

Similarly, aldosterone secretion can be stimulated directly by rising plasma potassium concentrations independent of the renin-angiotensin system.

Aldosterone

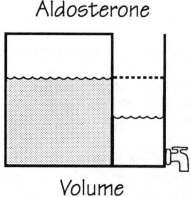

Volume

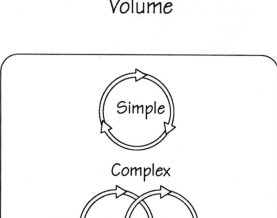

Simple

Complex

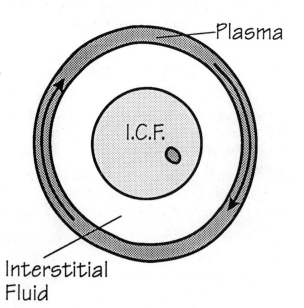

Plasma

I.C.F.

Interstitial
Fluid

In fact, these two hormones act together in a closely intergraded fashion in the control of volume and osmolality. However, for the moment, it is convenient to consider ADH as the "hormone of osmolality" and aldosterone as the "hormone of volume".

Others, such as atrial natriuretic peptides and the prostaglandins also have a role but their precise importance is not fully understood.

An important concept to grasp, is that the regulation of E.C.F. volume and osmolality is not related to a single feedback loop but rather to a number of interrelating and continuously operating feedback systems.

Neurogenic feedback loops tend to be rapid in their effect whereas humoral ones are slower. However, most loops combine both components even though one predominates.

Thus, beta adrenergic nerves are facilitators of renin release whilst epinephrine release from the adrenal medulla is part of the neurogenic response to a falling plasma volume.

Clinical Assessment of Changes in Fluid Compartments

Changes in the distribution of fluid volume between the major body compartments can be assessed by an observer at the bedside.

Because of its relative accessibility, the E.C.F. is open to clinical examination more readily than the I.C.F. which is "hidden" within the protective shell of the E.C.F.

Clinically the plasma compartment is the most accessible to assessment and even small changes can be detected.

The interstitial space is also accessible to the clinician but small changes may be very subtle and hard to detect. Large changes are usually very obvious.

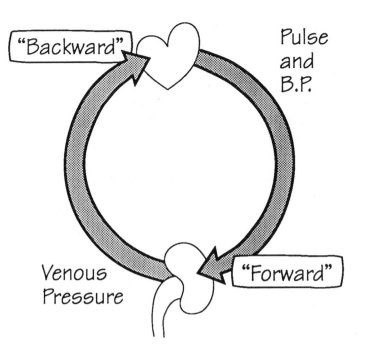

1. The Plasma Compartment

We have divided the plasma compartment into "backward" and "forward" components where changes in volume and flow go hand in hand.

"Forward" volume and flow are mirrored by the pulse and arterial pressure, whilst "backward" volume will be reflected by changes in venous pressure.

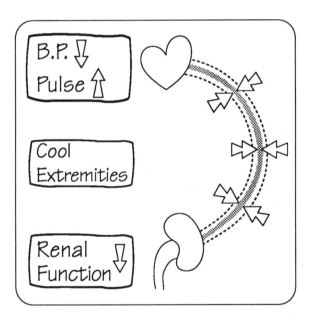

DIMINISHED "FORWARD" VOLUME AND FLOW

A low "forward" flow causes diminished peripheral circulation which is recognized by a fall in blood pressure and a compensatory rise in pulse rate.

Sometimes, the blood pressure is normal whilst lying but falls markedly on standing.

The hands and feet may be cold, often with peripheral cyanosis.

Poor perfusion of the kidneys may result in impaired renal function; poor cerebral perfusion may produce disturbed consciousness.

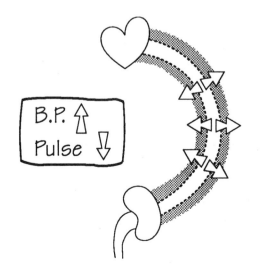

EXPANDED "FORWARD" VOLUME AND FLOW

An expanded "forward" flow will result in a rise in systemic arterial blood pressure and compensatory cardiac responses which include a reduced pulse rate.

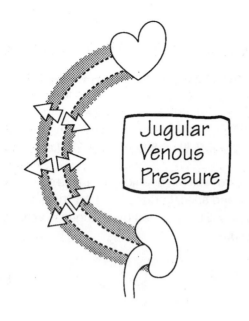

EXPANDED "BACKWARD" VOLUME AND FLOW

An expanded "backward" plasma volume will lead to elevated venous pressure seen in the jugular veins (with the patient propped up at 45°).

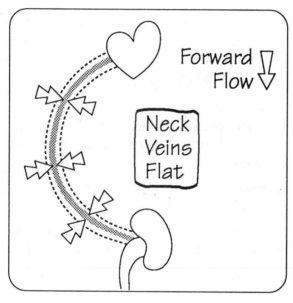

DIMINISHED "BACKWARD" VOLUME AND FLOW

A reduction of "backward" volume rapidly leads to a fall in cardiac filling and the signs of a low forward flow. In practice, therefore, there are few clinical features specific to a contracted venous volume, although the neck veins will not be visibly engorged.

Cardiologists refer to the backward volume as "pre-load" and the forward volume as "after load" and relate these terms to their effects on cardiac function. Thus, an increased pre-load results in greater diastolic filling while an increased after load demands greater ventricular contractile force.

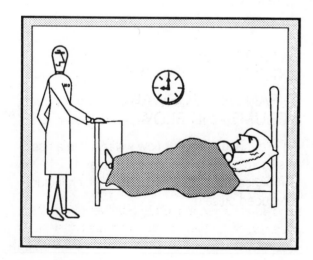

2. The Interstitial Compartment

The interstitial volume can also be assessed at the bedside and careful examination will be well worth the time.

Large changes are easy to detect but minor changes may be overlooked by a casual examination.

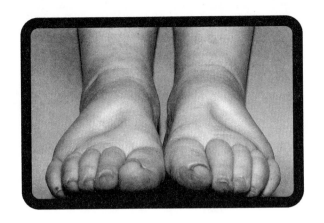

EXPANDED INTERSTITIAL VOLUME

An expanded interstitial volume will result in edema, revealed by the pitting produced by firm and sustained pressure with the thumb. Gravitational effects and the degree of laxity of subcutaneous tissues determine the distribution of generalized edema. Thus, it is most marked in the feet after a day of activity and in the face after a night's sleep.

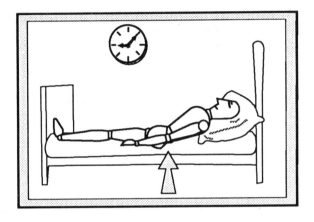

In a bedridden patient, edema will collect over the sacral area and may be missed by a hurried examination.

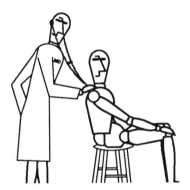

Interstitial edema in the pulmonary circulation is detected by hearing moist crepitations over the lung bases with a stethoscope.

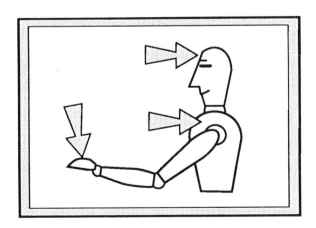

CONTRACTED INTERSTITIAL VOLUME

The signs of a contracted interstitial volume are sometimes subtle and not necessarily easy to detect.

Skin elasticity is reduced, best detected over a bony prominence where there is little subcutaneous fat; the forehead, the point of the shoulder, or the back of the hand are often used.

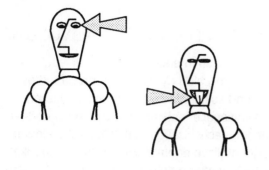

Other signs are dryness of mucous membranes, such as the tongue (unreliable in a mouth-breathing patient) and reduced eyeball tension (difficult to determine).

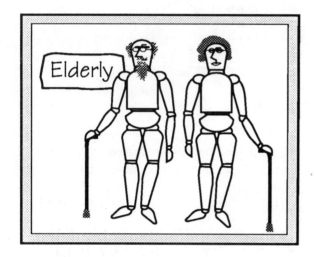

In the elderly, these signs may be difficult to assess, particularly because of the loss of elasticity of the skin with age. The complete absence of edema may be as important as the presence of reduced skin turgor in an elderly patient whose interstitial volume is reduced.

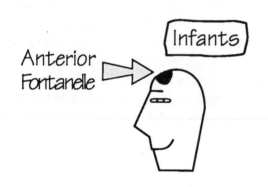

In the infant, the tension of the anterior fontanelle is a good indicator of interstitial volume. In contracted states, it will be more deeply depressed than usual, whilst in expanded states it may be slightly bulging.

Recent technical advances in intensive care medicine have seen the introduction of sophisticated electronic monitoring to the bedside.

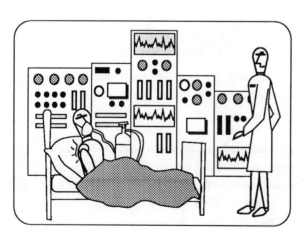

Direct measurement of intra-arterial pressure is commonplace.

Balloon-tipped catheters can be floated through the heart and out into the pulmonary circulation.

Cardiac output can be measured and indirect assessments of left atrial pressure can be made.

Techniques such as this have contributed much to the management of critically ill patients with disturbance of volume regulation.

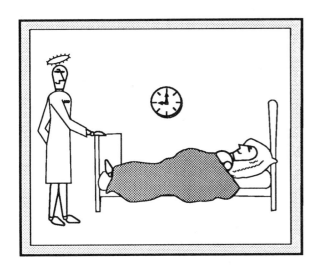

However, premature or inappropriate invasive monitoring can do more harm than good, and nothing can replace good clinical skills in the initial assessment and subsequent follow up of patients with volume problems.

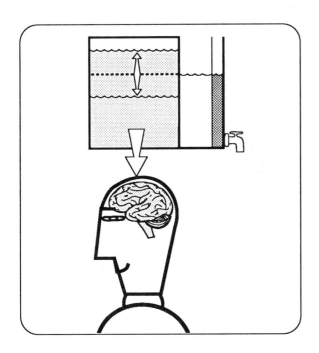

The Intra-cellular Compartment

Clinical assessment of the intracellular space is very difficult. The brain, because of its rigid bony constraints, is the organ whose function may reflect changes in the intracellular volume in a way that can be clinically apparent. Headache and confusion may occur with either expansion or contraction of the I.C.F. Expansion of the brain can only occur by herniation through the foramen magnum or in the presence of a hole in the skull.

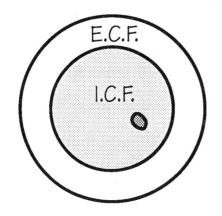

It is, of course, because the I.C.F. is surrounded by an E.C.F. "shell" that the I.C.F. is clinically inaccessible.

Clinical assessment of body fluids therefore means, for practical purposes, assessment of the E.C.F.

Chapter 5

Body Fluids in Abnormal States

Using the models built up in the previous chapters, it is now appropriate to discuss what happens when the system is stressed. The examples dealt with here are, of necessity, simplified, and provide only a skeleton upon which to hang the concepts of disordered regulation. Many details are left out in the interests of clarity, and not because they are unimportant.

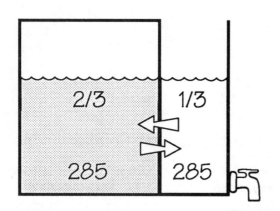

Remember that normally the relative volume of the intracellular and extracellular compartments in an adult is 2/3 : 1/3.

There is an osmotic balance between the two compartments both having an osmolality close to 285 milliosmoles per kilogram.

Sodium ions and chloride ions predominate in the E.C.F. and are the major determinants of its osmotic pressure.

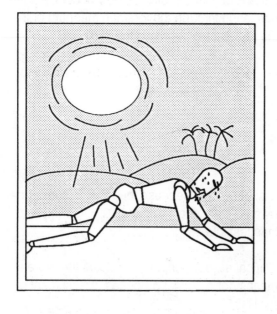

A Man in the Sahara

Now we can consider what would happen to this system if water was lost. Suppose we take the extreme example of an individual stranded in the Sahara Desert at high noon.

Water intake will be reduced to zero, but water loss will continue via the skin (as sweat) and the lungs. Water will also be lost as the obligatory solvent for those solutes that must be excreted in the urine. There will, of course, be a loss of sodium and chloride (as well as water) in the sweat, but to simplify the present example we may consider losses as being primarily water.

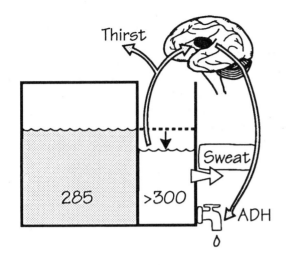

At first this will result in a loss of water from the E.C.F. and a rise in its sodium concentration and thus its osmolality. This will lead to thirst and the release of ADH which will minimize water losses by concentrating the urine maximally. Man is not well adapted to desert conditions and even under the severest stress, an adult will still excrete about 400 millilitres of water in the urine daily.

This continued loss of water from the E.C.F. leads to a rising sodium concentration, a rising osmolality, and a fall in its volume.

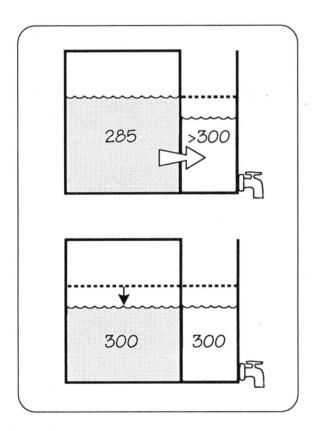

Normally, our traveller would drink water to correct matters but since there is no water, the osmotic gradient that has now been established between E.C.F. and I.C.F. leads to movement of water from the I.C.F. into the E.C.F. This movement will continue so long as an osmotic gradient exists between the two compartments.

With each upward step of E.C.F. osmolality there is a compensatory upward step in the I.C.F. osmolality. So long as no external water is available, this process will go on, resulting in a continuing fall of volume and rise of osmolality in both body compartments.

It is inevitable that in a system such as this, losses or gains of water are evenly distributed throughout total body water.

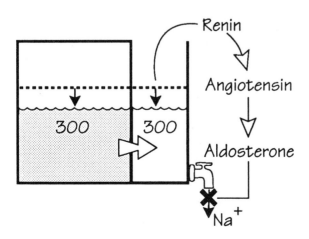

Because E.C.F. volume is reduced, the renin-angiotensin-aldosterone system will be activated and in addition to retaining water the kidney will also retain sodium which, in normal circumstances, would expand the plasma volume by retaining more water. In this case, however, no additional water is available and this compensation cannot occur.

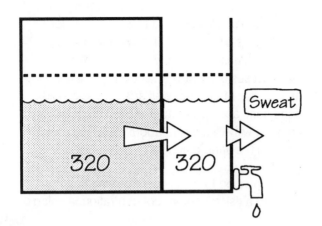

Each body compartment in our man in the desert becomes equally water-depleted. As the day gets hotter and the water gets scarcer, he continues to lose water. The osmolality of his E.C.F. goes on rising and so the osmolality of his I.C.F. also goes on rising. His fluid volumes gradually diminish, with equal distribution of volume contraction across all body compartments.

This will produce a dramatic clinical picture characterized by:

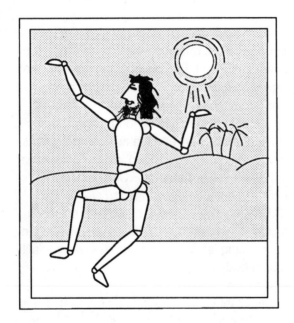

1. Signs of I.C.F. Volume Depletion

As time goes on there is continued intense stimulation of hypothalamic osmoreceptors. This produces intense thirst but there is no water available to correct it. Progressive shrinkage of the I.C.F. volume occurs. The effect of this is most obviously seen as a disturbance of function in the cells of the brain with the result that our deserted friend "goes mad with thirst".

2. Signs of E.C.F. Volume Depletion

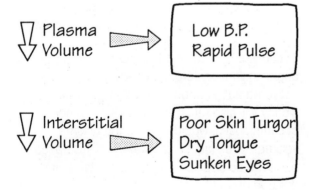

Physical examination at this time would make it apparent that both E.C.F. and I.C.F. had shrunk. There would be the signs of a reduced plasma volume, that is low blood pressure and rapid pulse. A reduction in interstitial volume would be indicated by poor skin turgor, dry tongue and sunken eyes. Because water has been lost, but only a relatively small amount of sodium and chloride, the serum sodium and chloride concentration will be markedly elevated.

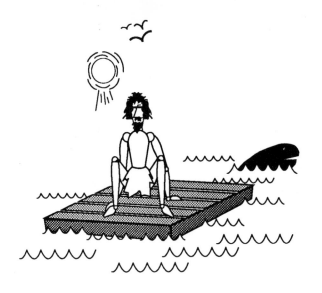

A Man in the Pacific Ocean

But now let's alter the situation and put him on a raft in the Pacific Ocean. Once again, there is exposure to heat and sunlight and still no fresh water is available but now he is surrounded by sea water with a sodium concentration of about 450 millimoles per litre.

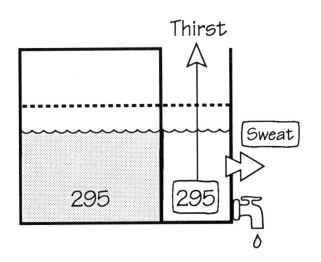

What happens at first is exactly what happened to the person in the Sahara Desert. An increasing osmolality develops in both compartments and a water deficit is spread throughout total body water.

This leads to thirst which may become severe enough to encourage the drinking of sea water in an attempt to relieve it.

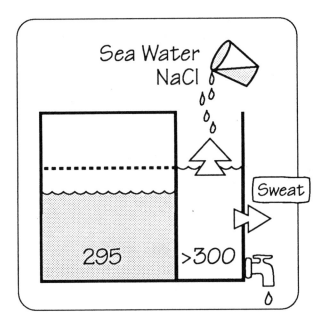

If sea water is drunk and the salt and water that is ingested is absorbed, it will stay in the E.C.F., increasing its volume and its osmolality.

It cannot be excreted because the normal human kidney is unable (even in the most favourable circumstances) to excrete urine with a sodium concentration above about 300 millimoles per litre. This means that to excrete 100 millilitres of sea water (equivalent to 450 millimolar sodium chloride), the kidney would have to excrete at least 150 millilitres of urine.

In other words, one could only drink sea water, and get away with it, so long as one had free access to a large supply of additional fresh water.

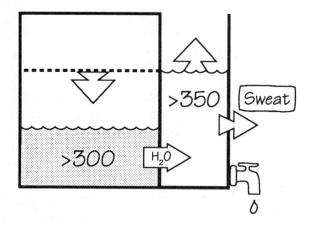

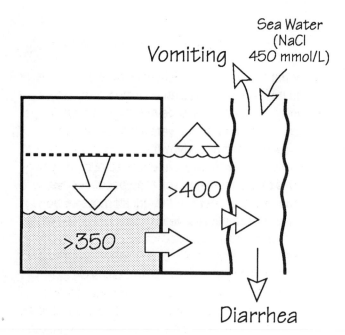

The E.C.F. will therefore become more hypertonic and its volume will tend to increase at the expense of the I.C.F.

The osmotic gradient between the two compartments results in continued movement of water out of the cells, thus reducing I.C.F. volume and increasing I.C.F. osmolality to match the osmolality of E.C.F.

In reality other factors complicate this theoretical picture. For example:

1) Sea water contains magnesium ions which will induce diarrhea and vomiting, which deplete E.C.F. volume.

2) Hypertonic fluid in the intestine will effectively suck water directly out of the E.C.F. since they communicate intimately (see page 3).

Regardless of the resulting degree and the direction of change in E.C.F. volume, there is inexorable and progressive intra-cellular dehydration as the E.C.F. osmolality rises.

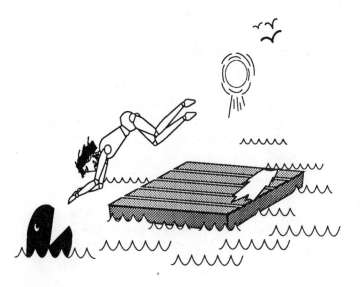

The ultimate disturbances of water distribution and volume regulation in individuals who drink sea water are more dramatic and more rapid than those occurring in those who resist the drive to drink. The rapid cellular dehydration leads to rapid and severe disturbances of intracerebral function and an earlier departure!

These examples have been extreme, and for many of us entirely theoretical, but they have been used to make a point. There are, however, more common pathological situations where the same mechanisms operate, and two brief examples will be given here.

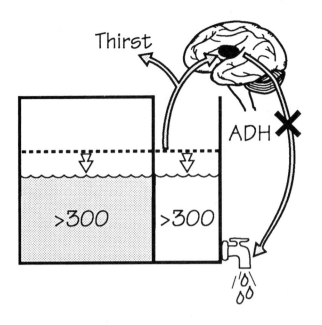

1. Patients with Diabetes Insipidus

Patients with a fracture to the base of the skull and damage to the hypothalamus may lose the ability to produce ADH and therefore cannot control water loss from the kidney.

If their level of consciousness becomes disturbed and they cannot respond to thirst, they will become water depleted just as surely as if they were in the desert with no water. This clinical picture is called "Diabetes Insipidus".

2. An Unconscious Patient

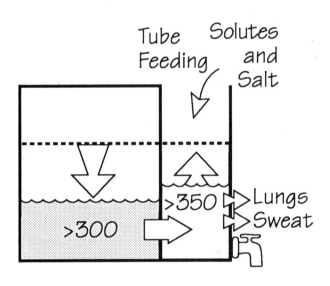

Another example is patients who are unconscious and have a tracheostomy and a fever. Increased losses of water from the lungs and from increased sweating may be underestimated. Since they cannot complain of thirst (because they are unconscious), they may become deprived of water just as surely as our friend in the desert. Their plight may not be recognized until the increased concentration of solutes (particularly sodium) is noted in their blood. If the problem of their inadequate water intake is compounded by an increase of the solute load by tube feeding with high calorie, low volume food concentrates, they may closely approximate the conditions of our shipwrecked mariner who drinks hypertonic sea water.

Sodium, Water and Volume

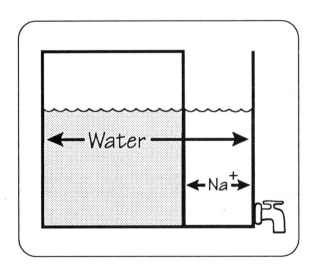

These situations demonstrate how close is the link between sodium and water in determining the volume of intracellular and extracellular spaces.

1) Water is distributed across all body compartments.

2) Sodium is confined to the E.C.F. and by its osmotic effect determines the volume of the E.C.F.

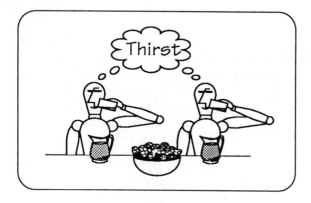

In a healthy individual any excess of sodium that is ingested will result in a change in osmolality, thirst, subsequent drinking, and, finally, expansion of the E.C.F. As an example, we are all familiar with being thirsty after a salty meal, and it is no accident that whilst the salted peanuts are free, the thirst that they produce may be expensive!

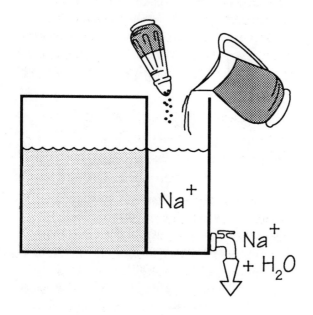

In a normal subject, this volume expansion is registered by volume receptors, resulting in reduced secretion of aldosterone (and ADH) which limit renal tubular absorption of filtered sodium and water until the excess has been excreted. In a normal subject with a healthy heart and kidneys, it is almost impossible to overload the E.C.F. by eating salt and drinking water.

However, if the heart is not normal, or if volume regulation in the E.C.F. is disturbed, this normal response will be incomplete.

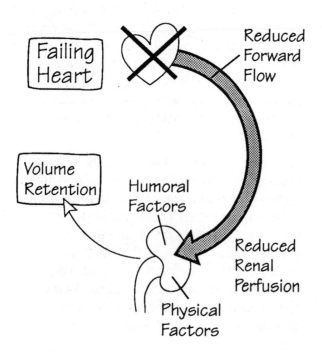

Heart Failure

Two more clinical examples will demonstrate the problems that may result.

The first example is someone with heart failure. The initial problem here is that the "effective forward blood flow" is reduced. The heart cannot pump adequately, and so the effective arterial volume and flow are reduced.

This leads to under-perfusion of the kidney and a series of responses which result in retention of sodium and water by the renal tubule. These responses include physical factors within the kidney and humoral factors acting on renal perfusion and renal tubular function. (See Chapter 6).

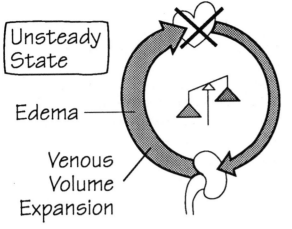

Unsteady
State

Edema

Venous
Volume
Expansion

The retention of sodium and water lead to expansion of the plasma volume, but if the heart is failing as a pump it cannot distribute the added volume from the "backward" to the "forward" halves of the circulation.

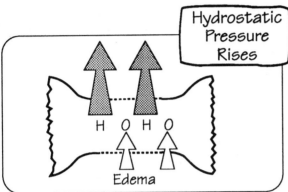

Hydrostatic
Pressure
Rises

H O H O

Edema

As a result, the hydrostatic pressure at the venous end of the capillaries rises, and the Starling hypothesis (relating to fluid movements in and out of the capillaries) tells us that volume will shift out of the plasma compartment into the interstitial space.

And so edema occurs, and continues to get worse if the heart cannot respond to increased venous filling by increasing its output.

The expanded venous volume and increased venous return to the heart stretch the cardiac muscle fibres and this may result in improved cardiac output (Starling's Law of the heart). This can result in a new steady state where forward flow improves because of expansion of venous volume ("compensated" heart failure).

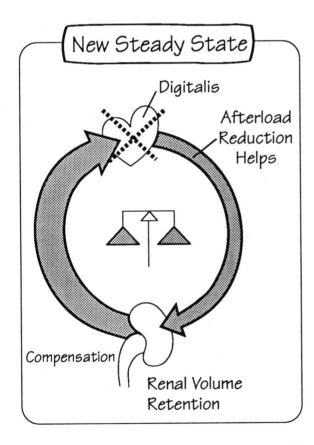

New Steady State

Digitalis

Afterload
Reduction
Helps

Compensation

Renal Volume
Retention

This description of cardiac failure is greatly simplified, but does emphasize the importance of renal responses in the compensation for a failing heart by the retention of salt and water. So long as cardiac function improves in response to volume loading, this compensatory response is to the benefit of the whole organism.

Effective treatment aims at improving the ability of the heart to pump volume forward. Lowering systemic arterial resistance, using vasodilators ("after-load reduction") or the use of Digoxin may both achieve this effect. Diuretics block retention of volume by the kidney and may therefore block the compensation that was described in the previous paragraph; for this reason diuretics are not necessarily the appropriate first step at therapy.

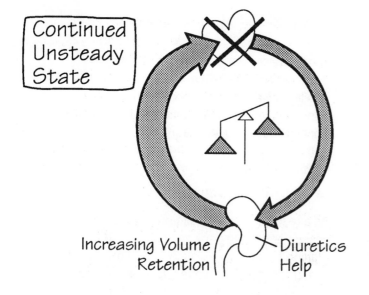

Increasing Volume Retention — Diuretics Help

The improved cardiac output resulting from increased filling volume of the heart and predicted by Starling's Law, occurs up to a point. Beyond that point, however, further increases of volume "behind the heart" do not produce further increase in output, and as the heart dilates, output may even fall.

In this situation, the renal retention of salt and water compounds the initial problem of the failing heart, and far from being a compensation becomes an aggravating factor that perpetuates a deteriorating "unsteady state". Reduction of volume load with diuretics now becomes a priority of treatment.

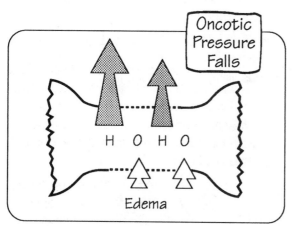

Oncotic Pressure Falls

H O H O

Edema

Hypoalbuminemia

Another clinical example of disordered regulation of the E.C.F. is seen when the serum albumin is reduced, such as by failure to synthesize it in liver disease. In this case, effective blood volume is reduced as fluid leaks out of the capillaries into the interstitial space because of a reduction of colloid osmotic pressure rather than because of a rising hydrostatic pressure.

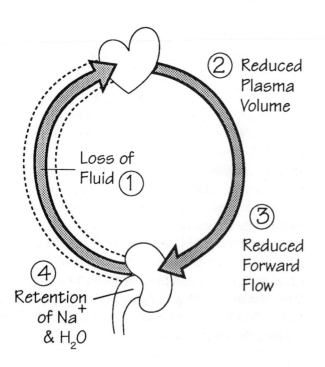

② Reduced Plasma Volume

Loss of Fluid ①

③ Reduced Forward Flow

④ Retention of Na^+ & H_2O

The kidney registers this as if it represented an overall reduction of plasma flow, and so the same changes that occurred in heart failure are set in motion. These result in retention of sodium and water, and the exaggeration of edema which continues to accumulate as long as the receptors in the kidney and elsewhere register a "volume deficit".

Thus, salt and water are continually retained and continue to leak out into the interstitial space as long as the plasma albumin level remains inadequate.

Because the heart is healthy, the plasma volume and flow are not "asymmetrical" as in heart failure, and the reduction in volume is on both the arterial and venous sides of the circulation.

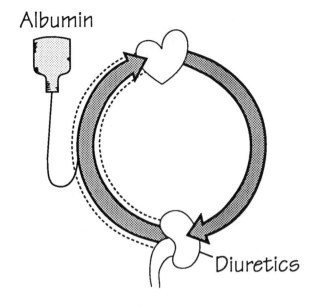

Albumin

Diuretics

In this example, diuretics may improve the edema by blocking retention of salt and water, but in doing so they are blocking the response to a pathological stimulus and not correcting its cause. In fact, potent diuretics, by blocking volume retention, may actually reduce plasma volume and flow further, and thus make the situation worse by exaggerating the abnormality that started the volume retention at the outset.

Infusing albumin is obviously the "physiologically appropriate" first line of treatment; just as in treating heart failure with digitalis the need for diuretics may be eliminated by correcting the primary cause of the volume retention.

Two Final Concepts

1) In these examples of disorders of body fluid regulation, it should be clear to the reader that volume within the E.C.F. is tightly linked to the loss or gain of sodium which, by its osmotic effects, determines how much water will enter or leave the E.C.F.

The regulation of volume and the regulation of sodium cannot be separated in attempts to understand the regulation of the E.C.F. and by inference the I.C.F. as well.

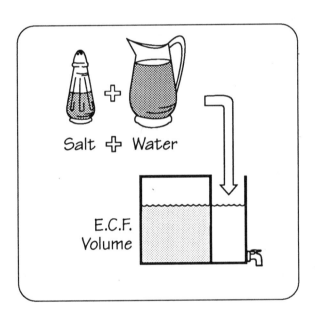

Salt ✚ Water

E.C.F. Volume

2) In any consideration of the plasma compartment, it will be apparent that volume, flow and pressure are intimately related. Thus it is that the flow into the heart balances the flow out of the heart, although volume and pressure differ greatly between veins and arteries. Stimuli which result in volume retention by the kidney may be triggered by sensors that respond to pressure and flow (such as the juxtaglomerular apparatus in the kidney). Similarly, stimulation of sensors for volume in the great veins and right side of the heart may result in an increase of arterial pressure and flow. Any change in one of these factors will modify the other two and this is a fact of life in the plasma compartment.

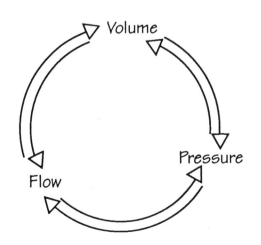

Volume

Flow

Pressure

Chapter 6

The Regulation of Sodium

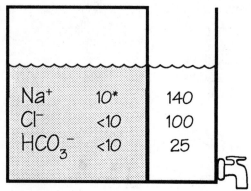

*All values are mmol/L

Na⁺	10*	140
Cl⁻	<10	100
HCO₃⁻	<10	25

The major regulator of body sodium is the kidney. Since sodium is the major determinant of E.C.F. volume, the kidney is therefore the major regulator of E.C.F. volume.

Sodium, and its accompanying anions, chloride and bicarbonate, are the major osmotically active particles in the E.C.F. None of them is present within the cells to any major extent.

This partition depends upon an active pump in the walls of all cells. Using energy stored in adenosine-triphosphate (ATP) and releasing it via an ATP-ase the cells pump out the sodium that leaks in and exchange it for potassium that leaks out.

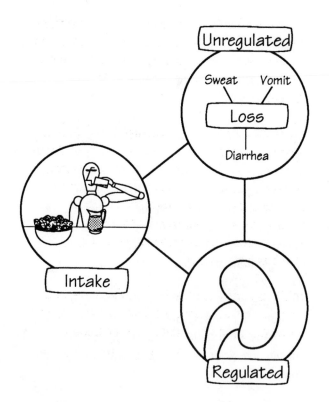

Sodium Balance

In normal health, sodium enters the body only by eating and drinking and the balance between intake and output ensures stable E.C.F. volume.

Significant losses, in the stool or by vomiting, cannot be regulated and are always pathological. Losses by sweating are dependent upon environmental factors and are open to relatively little regulation.

The only route of loss that can be regulated with precision is via the urine. Here we will look at this mechanism in more detail and consider the role of the kidney in states of sodium retention or loss.

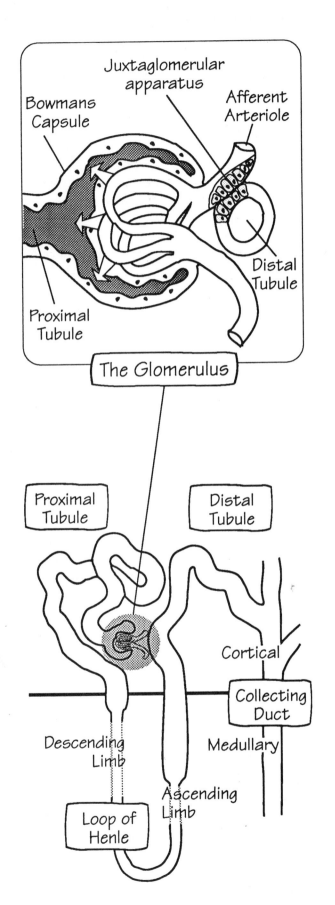

Juxtaglomerular apparatus

Bowmans Capsule

Afferent Arteriole

Distal Tubule

Proximal Tubule

The Glomerulus

Proximal Tubule

Distal Tubule

Cortical

Collecting Duct

Medullary

Descending Limb

Ascending Limb

Loop of Henle

The Nephron

The nephron is the unit of function in the kidney, and within the nephron lie the mechanisms which allow the precise regulation of the sodium content of the E.C.F.

Each kidney contains approximately a million of these units, in which structure and function are indivisible. Filtration at the glomerulus delivers fluid to the tubule where its composition is modified by reabsorption, secretion or a combination of the two.

Glomerular Filtration

Glomerular filtration occurs as hydrostatic pressure forces fluid out of the glomerular capillaries into the urinary space. This effect is modified by the oncotic pressure of the plasma proteins and depends upon the permeability of the capillary wall in the glomerulus.

The glomerular filtrate is essentially an ultrafiltrate of plasma and it enters a tubule which is long and follows a winding course until it joins with other tubules forming the collecting ducts in the medullary papilla.

The schematic tubule shown here is subdivided into four major segments and each of them shows specialization of function. After forming the loop of Henle the ascending tubule comes back to nestle close to its parent glomerulus forming the juxtaglomerular apparatus. This provides a point at which feedback between tubule and glomerulus can occur.

This is also the site of renin production. Renin is an important regulator of sodium reabsorption and will be discussed in greater detail on page 71.

61

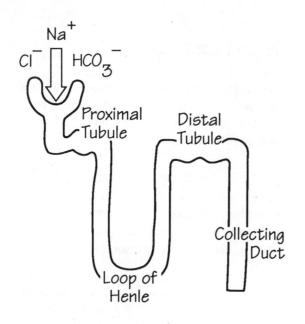

Any diagrammatic representation of the nephron is, of course, greatly simplified. In future pages the stylized nephron shown here will be used.

In the absence of a barrier to filtration, and in the presence of relatively high serum concentrations, sodium, chloride, and bicarbonate will pass rapidly into the glomerular filtrate.

Tubular Reabsorption

Knowing the glomerular filtration rate, it is easy to calculate the filtered load which can then be compared to the amount appearing in the final urine.

As is shown in this table, the amount of water and ions which are filtered every day is very large, but the efficiency with which they can be reabsorbed on their way down the tubule is remarkable.

	Amt. Filtered Per Day	Amt. Excreted Per Day	% Reabsorbed Per Day
Sodium	25,000 mmol	100 mmol	99.6%
Chloride	18,000 mmol	100 mmol	99.5%
Bicarbonate	5,000 mmol	Nil	100%
Potassium	700 mmol	50 mmol	93.0%
Water	180L	1L	99.4%

These figures are based upon a normal adult on a normal diet. If the same individual is put on a sodium-free diet the daily urine sodium losses will fall to only two or three millimoles, increasing the completeness of sodium reabsorption to very nearly 100%.

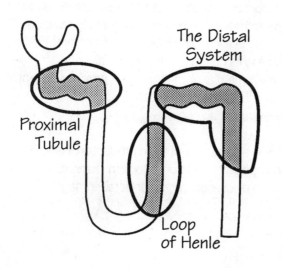

Obviously, the kidney has a very well developed ability to recapture and conserve filtered sodium. Quantitatively, most of this is reabsorbed in the proximal tubule but more distal sites of absorption are qualitatively just as important. Reabsorption at the three sites shown in this "stylized" nephron will now be reviewed.

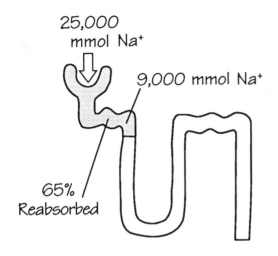

25,000
mmol Na⁺

9,000 mmol Na⁺

65%
Reabsorbed

The Proximal Tubule

About 65% of the filtered load can be reabsorbed in this segment of the nephron, all of it by a process involving active transport of sodium from the tubular fluid, through the tubular cells and out into the peritubular space where it can enter the peritubular capillary network. Of the 25,000 millimoles filtered per day, only about 9,000 still remain by the time the tubular fluid reaches the beginning of the loop of Henle.

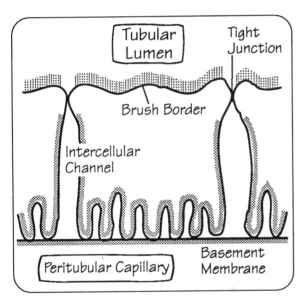

Tubular Lumen

Tight Junction

Brush Border

Intercellular Channel

Peritubular Capillary

Basement Membrane

The cells concerned in this reabsorptive process line the proximal tubule and rest on a basement membrane which separates them from the peritubular interstitial space. The cells have basal infoldings around which are many mitochondria. The luminal border of the cells has a surface covered with projecting microvilli which increase its area and is seen as a "brush border" under the light microscope.

In between the cells are intercellular channels, but the communication between these channels and the lining of the tubule is blocked by a "tight" junction. In the proximal tubule, the tight junction is in fact a fairly leaky area through which significant amounts of ions and fluid can pass.

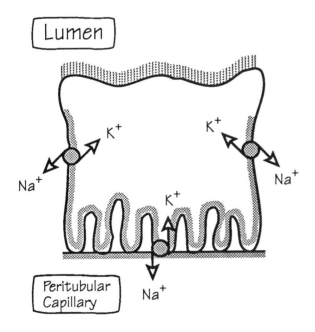

Lumen

K⁺

K⁺

Na⁺

Na⁺

K⁺

Na⁺

Peritubular Capillary

The recovery of sodium, its accompanying anions and water, from the glomerular filtrate is an energy requiring process. The energy is provided by the activity of membrane bound ATP-ase which releases energy from ATP to power a pump which pushes sodium out of the tubular cell in exchange for returning potassium to the cell. The effect of the pump is to keep the cell sodium at a low level which then provides an environment where sodium can move from the lumen into the cell by processes that are essentially passive. The pump operates across the base of the cell and also across its lateral walls into the intercellular spaces. These areas are collectively called "the basolateral membrane".

There is no such pump at the luminal border of the cell, and in subsequent diagrams in the next few pages, the active sodium/potassium pump will be designated by a shaded circle.

63

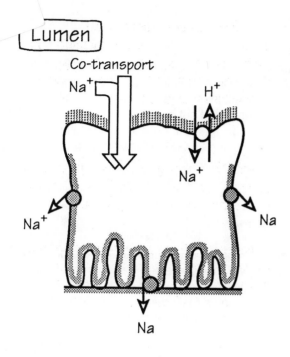

Lumen

Co-transport

Sodium enters the cell from the lumen by two pathways.

1) By co-transport using a carrier which links sodium transport to the transport of amino acids, glucose or phosphate.

2) By means of exchange transport with hydrogen ion. This "anti- porter" moves hydrogen ion out of the cell in a linkage with sodium moving into the cell.

Having entered the cell, the sodium can then move across the basolateral membrane by the activity of the active pump.

The osmotic gradient produced by these ionic movements carries water across the cell as well.

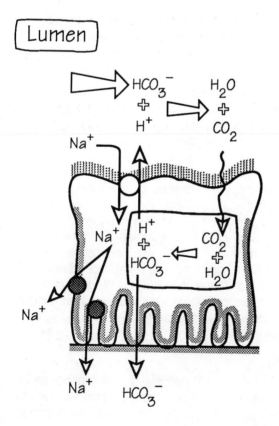

Lumen

Hydrogen ion that enters the antiporter system is manufactured within the cell from carbon dioxide and water which produces hydrogen ion and bicarbonate.

The enzyme carbonic anhydrase is important as a catalyst of this reaction.

Once the hydrogen ion has entered the lumen the following events occur:

1) Bicarbonate in the filtrate is trapped and promptly turned into CO_2 and water with the aid of Carbonic Anhydrase in the brush border. At the same time, freshly made bicarbonate crosses the basolateral membrane into the interstitial space. The CO_2 in the lumen diffuses back into the cell to promote further production of bicarbonate. This process is the equivalent of reabsorption of bicarbonate.

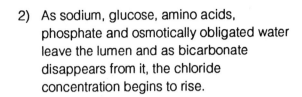

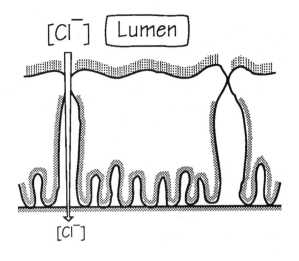

2) As sodium, glucose, amino acids, phosphate and osmotically obligated water leave the lumen and as bicarbonate disappears from it, the chloride concentration begins to rise.

3) Chloride now moves down its concentration gradient from the lumen into the interstitial space, predominately via a paracellular pathway.

At no time are there any major gradients of electrical potential across the cell during this process.

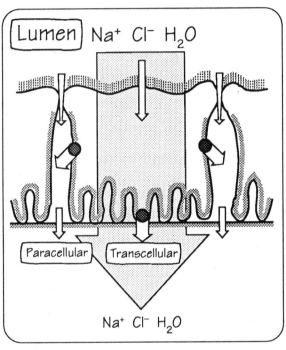

The end result, in the proximal tubule, is the transport of isotonic sodium chloride from lumen to E.C.F. Along with it goes co-transported solutes and what amounts to the "reabsorption" of bicarbonate from the proximal tubular fluid.

The massive amounts of sodium and water reabsorbed in the proximal system (see the table on page 62) is all powered via the energy of the sodium pump in the basolateral membrane and involves the movement of sodium, chloride and water through both transcellular and paracellular pathways.

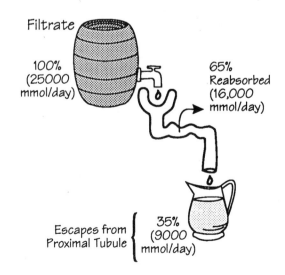

At the end of the proximal tubule about 65% of the filtered sodium, water and chloride has been reabsorbed, but the fluid in the tubular lumen remains isotonic as it enters the loop of Henle, where a second phase of sodium recovery occurs.

65

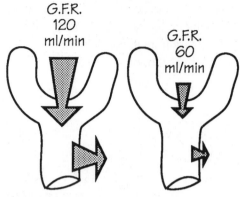

G.F.R.
120
ml/min

G.F.R.
60
ml/min

"Glomerular Tubular Balance"

Regulation of Proximal Reabsorption

There is a linkage between glomerular filtration rate (G.F.R.) and tubular reabsorption. Experiment has shown that there is a continuing relationship, in normal physiologic situations between G.F.R. and reabsorption. The less filtered, the less reabsorbed, and conversely the more filtered, the more reabsorbed. Expressed in another way, the fraction of filtrate reabsorbed remains constant as the G.F.R. changes. This behaviour has been called "glomerular tubular balance".

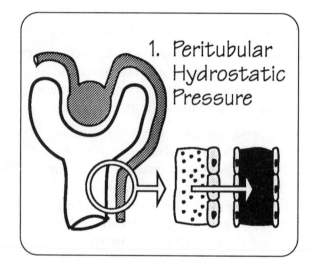

1. Peritubular Hydrostatic Pressure

This relationship between G.F.R. and tubular reabsorption has been explained by a number of theories. Amongst these, two factors will be mentioned: they depend upon the fact that the capillary network carrying blood around the proximal tubule is, in fact, in direct continuity with the efferent arteriole, so that blood from the glomerular tuft then courses around its own proximal tubule. Clearly, the more plasma that is filtered, the more the hydrostatic pressure in the efferent arteriole and the peritubular capillaries into which it empties will tend to fall. Thus the tendency for salt and water to leave the tubule and pass back into the peritubular capillaries, will be greater if the G.F.R. is increased.

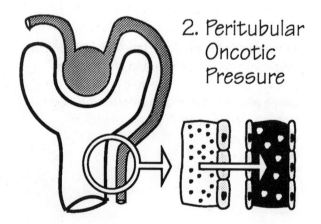

2. Peritubular Oncotic Pressure

In a similar manner, the greater the filtration at the glomerulus, the more will the plasma proteins be concentrated by loss of water and diffusible solutes. Thus the effective osmotic pressure due to the plasma proteins will increase in the peritubular capillaries. This will also favour movement of sodium and water out of the tubule at a rate which increases with increasing filtration.

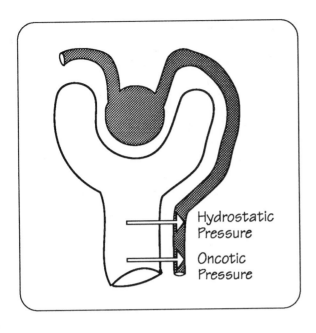

Hydrostatic Pressure

Oncotic Pressure

Third Factor

Thus two mechanisms, both relating to physical characteristics of peritubular fluid and dependent upon the renal vascular architecture, will favour a positive relationship between the G.F.R. and proximal tubular reabsorption.

The supposition that humoral agents might be effective in modulating proximal tubular sodium reabsorption led to the term "third factor" being coined. This term referred to factors other than 1) Changing G.F.R. and 2) Aldosterone (which, of course, acts on the distal tubule).

A prolonged search has led to no specific conclusions. The humoral agents that have surfaced during this search probably do not act on the proximal tubule but may act on the glomerular filtration rate. They include: Atrial natriuretic peptides and Prostaglandins

There still remains the possibility of an endogenous inhibitor of proximal tubular ATP-ase (perhaps produced by the hypothalamus) but this remains unproven.

The Loop of Henle

The second site in the tubule for sodium reabsorption is the loop of Henle. Only about 25% of the total load is reabsorbed here, but it is a critical 25% because on it depends the effectiveness of the countercurrent system for water conservation. This will be discussed in more detail in Chapter 7.

This fragment of sodium transport probably remains constant in most physiologic situations. It can, however, be influenced by a group of potent diuretic drugs which block ionic transport at this site. For this reason, they are called "loop diuretics" and examples are furosemide and ethacrynic acid. The major site of sodium transport is in the thick ascending limb of the loop and once again, the energy for transport is provided by the basolateral sodium pump which maintains a low intracellular sodium concentration.

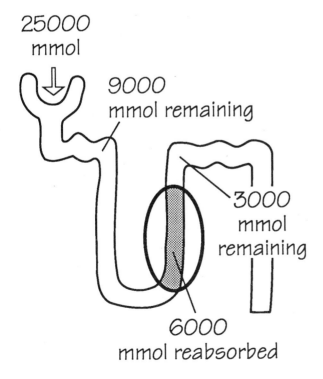

25000 mmol

9000 mmol remaining

3000 mmol remaining

6000 mmol reabsorbed

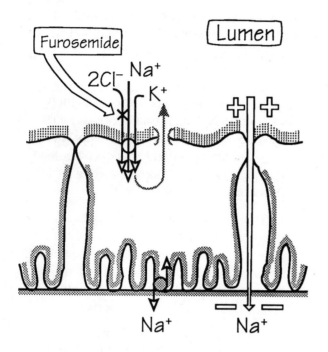

Sodium enters the luminal membrane through a carrier which links the transport of one sodium ion, one potassium ion and two chloride ions. The affinity of the carrier for sodium is very high and the availability of chloride is the rate-limiting factor. Loop diuretics appear to block the process by competing for chloride at the carrier.

Potassium ions are not rate-limiting because there is continuous recycling of potassium through a specific channel in the luminal membrane so that potassium is continually available to activate the carrier.

This movement of potassium into the lumen creates a lumen positive potential difference and this allows the passive movement of positively charged ions (such as sodium, calcium and magnesium) through the paracellular route.

The role of this mechanism in generating the energy for free water reabsorption will be discussed in Chapter 7.

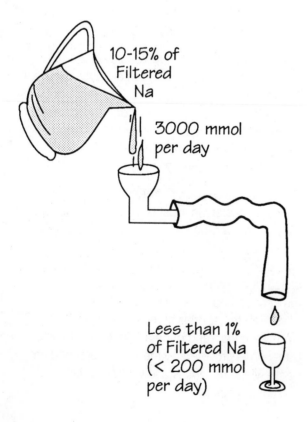

The Distal System

Beyond the loop of Henle the "distal system" can be divided into a number of parts. These include 1) the distal convoluted tubule 2) the connecting segment 3) the cortical collecting tubule and 4) the medullary collecting tubule.

While these segments are differentiated on the basis of differences in function, it is reasonable to simplify this somewhat and look at the distal system in relation to two mechanisms of sodium reabsorption.

About 10-15% of filtered sodium reaches the distal system and there is a potential for almost complete reabsorption of all the sodium that enters it. In conditions of profound sodium restriction, sodium loss in the urine can be reduced to a few millimoles a day.

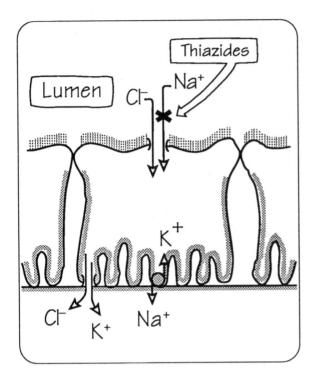

1. The Distal Convoluted Tubule

About 5% of filtered sodium is reabsorbed here and once again the sodium/potassium pump in the basolateral membrane provides the energy to keep the cell sodium at a low level. Sodium then enters the luminal membrane via a sodium and chloride co-transport system. This differs from the system in the ascending limb of the loop of Henle in that potassium is not a part of the luminal transport system and this is the area where thiazide diuretics inhibit sodium chloride reabsorption.

2. The Cortical Collecting Duct

In this segment, there are two types of cells. These are:

1) The principal cells
   and
2) The intercalated cells

Two-thirds of the cells are principal cells and are related to sodium transport. The remaining one third are intercalated cells and perform no sodium transporting function, being related to hydrogen ion transport.

In the principal cells, there is once again an active basolateral sodium pump and sodium enters on the luminal side by specific sodium channels. This movement of positive ions across the membrane creates a potential which is lumen negative and this allows the secretion of potassium down its concentration gradient through potassium channels. An alternative is the passage of chloride through the paracellular pathway.

This part of the reabsorptive system is regulated by aldosterone which increases the number of sodium channels available on the luminal surface.

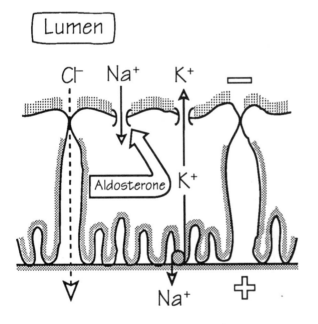

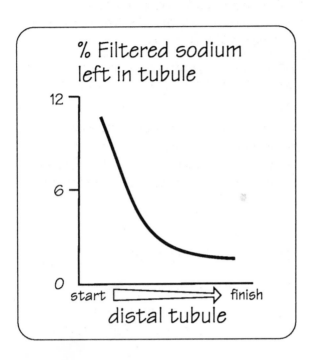

% Filtered sodium left in tubule

The Distal System - Regulation

The end result of the processes in the distal system allows the almost complete disappearance of sodium from the tubular fluid by the time it reaches the renal pelvis.

The regulation of sodium reabsorption here is carried out by hormonal mechanisms whose final messenger is the steroid hormone aldosterone.

The first step in this regulation is the release of a protein called renin from granules in the wall of the afferent arteriole where it becomes closely related to the distal tubule of its own nephron.

The cells in the tubule wall at this point are closely applied to the arteriolar wall and are called the "macular densa". This area is collectively called the "juxtaglomerular apparatus".

Sensors in the wall of the afferent arteriole respond to changes in blood pressure and flow which may result from the loss or gain of sodium from the E.C.F.

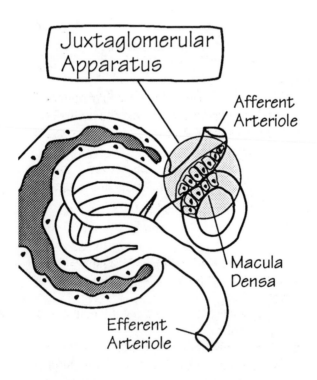

Renin release from the juxtaglomerular apparatus is promoted by three mechanisms.

1) Stimulation of stretch receptors in the afferent arteriolar wall.

2) Stimulation of cardiac and arterial baroreceptors which lead to renin release via adrenergic nerves.

3) Stimulation of the cells in the macula densa by a fall in luminal chloride delivery.

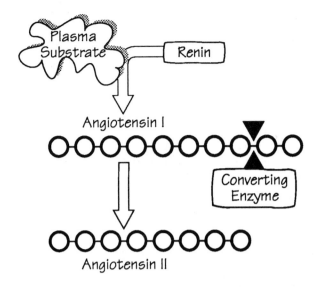

Angiotensin I

Converting Enzyme

Angiotensin II

Renin then acts on a protein substrate (angiotensinogen) made in the liver to release the decapeptide angiotensin I.

Finally, converting enzyme removes two amino acids from angiotensin I to produce angiotensin II.

Converting enzyme is present in highest concentration in the lungs. However, all components of the renin-angiotensin system are present in vascular endothelium including the glomerulus.

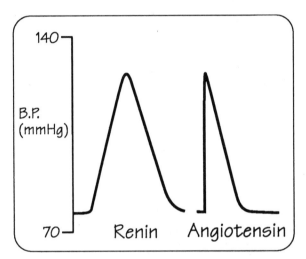

Effects of Angiotensin II

Angiotensin II has two systemic effects.

1) The first is to raise the blood pressure by increasing the systemic arteriolar resistance. In an animal model, the effects of infusing angiotensin II are potent and immediate. The effects of infusing renin are delayed because the enzymatic steps needed to release angiotensin II take a finite amount of time.

2) The second effect is to promote the reabsorption of sodium from the tubule by two separate actions.
a) The most important is by stimulating the release of aldosterone from the cortex of the adrenal gland. This leads to distal sodium reabsorption.
b) By directly increasing the activity of the sodium-hydrogen antiporter in the luminal membrane of the proximal tubule.

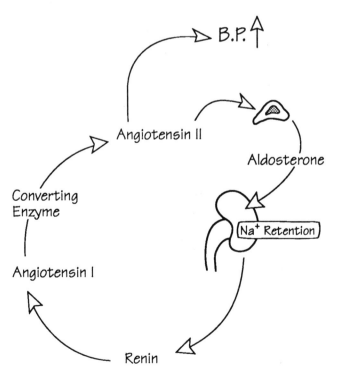

There are also local actions of angiotensin II relating to the regulation of glomerular filtration rate and these include:
a) Constriction of the efferent arteriole of the glomerulus.
b) The release of prostaglandins which are vasodilator probably to the afferent arteriole.
c) A contraction of the mesangial cells which may reduce the surface area of the glomerulus.

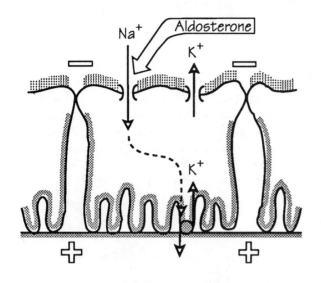

Aldosterone activates sodium reabsorption in the collecting duct by increasing the number of channels available for sodium movement across the luminal membrane. This increased entry of sodium drives the sodium pump to expel more sodium across the basolateral membrane and as this occurs there is a greater efflux of potassium across the luminal membrane down the electrical gradient generated by sodium movement. The end result is an increased reabsorption of sodium and an increased secretion of potassium.

Aldosterone also acts upon sodium and potassium transport in the colon, sweat glands and salivary glands, but these actions are much less impressive then its action on the renal tubule.

Proximal Tubule

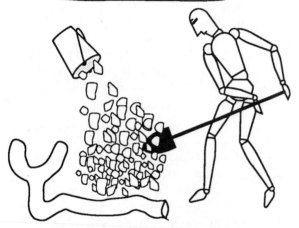

Bulk of the work load

In Summary...

Most of the filtered sodium is reabsorbed in the proximal tubule. The degree of this reabsorption is related to the G.F.R., the peritubular physical environment and perhaps humoral factors although these are not fully clarified. 65% of filtered sodium is reabsorbed proximally leaving the remainder to enter the loop of Henle.

In the loop of Henle reabsorption is probably more or less constant and represents perhaps 25% of the filtered load.

Distal Tubule

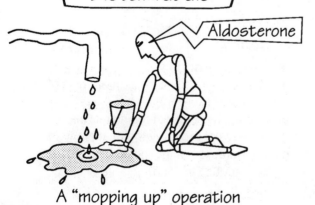

A "mopping up" operation

In the distal tubule, the amount of sodium reabsorbed is not nearly so large, but the completeness of its reabsorption in times of stress may be extreme.

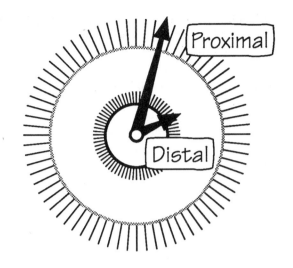

The major regulator of sodium reabsorption at this site is aldosterone. Proximal regulation of sodium recovery may be considered as the "coarse tuning" of the system whilst the more accurate "fine tuning" takes place in the distal system.

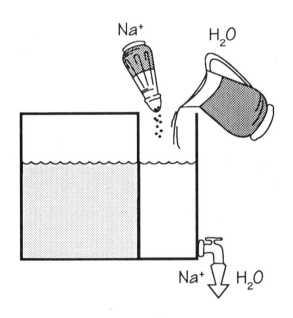

Clinical Examples of Disordered Sodium Handling

Losses or gains of sodium (and accompanying anions) is usually associated with equivalent losses or gains of water. In most instances losses or gains are isotonic.

Because of this, retention or loss of sodium is indicated by changes in the volume of the E.C.F. and not by changes in the concentration of sodium in the E.C.F.

This means that the plasma sodium concentration is a poor indicator of the amount of sodium in the body.

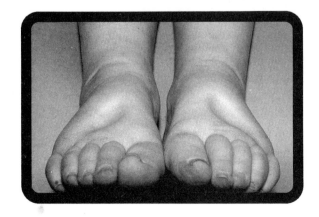

Sodium Retention - Edema

The cardinal sign of sodium retention is generalized edema. Sodium cannot be retained without the inevitable retention of water, but because sodium remains in the E.C.F., it is this compartment that expands.

Edema is a sign of interstitial fluid expansion and may occur with or without demonstrable expansion of the plasma volume.

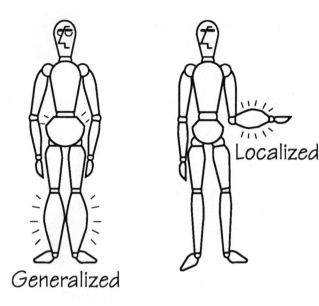

Generalized

Localized

Edema is not always generalized. It may be localized, and in such cases does not represent a primary disorder of sodium metabolism. Localized edema implies one of the following mechanisms.

1) Venous obstruction

2) Capillary wall damage, usually due to inflammation

3) Lymphatic obstruction (in which case the edema may be non-pitting).

Subsequent discussion will confine itself to the issue of generalized edema.

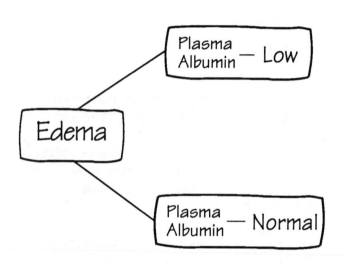

Edema → Plasma Albumin — Low

Edema → Plasma Albumin — Normal

Generalized edema implies an overall change in the osmotic or hydrostatic events in the capillary bed throughout the body and may be associated with:

1) A reduced plasma albumin level or

2) A normal plasma albumin level

Low Plasma Albumin

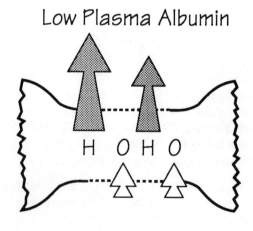

H O H O

1. Edema With a Low Plasma Albumin

If the albumin level is reduced, the mechanism of the edema is a reduced oncotic pressure in the capillaries and a consequent leak of fluid out of the plasma space into the interstitial compartment, with a resulting diminution of plasma volume.

This, of course, matches the predictions of the Starling hypothesis.

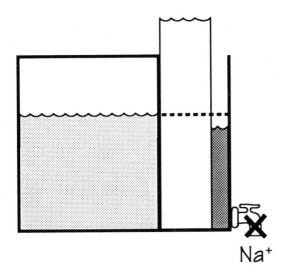

Since the plasma volume is relatively reduced, the neck veins are not engorged and the blood pressure is not elevated.

Since effective renal blood flow is also relatively reduced, sodium retention will occur due to direct and indirect (hormone dependent) renal mechanisms.

Because of the low plasma oncotic pressure, however, the retained sodium and water continue to move out into the interstitial space increasing interstitial edema without plasma volume expansion. So long as the plasma albumin concentration remains low, there will be an imbalance of volume distribution in the E.C.F. favouring interstitial expansion.

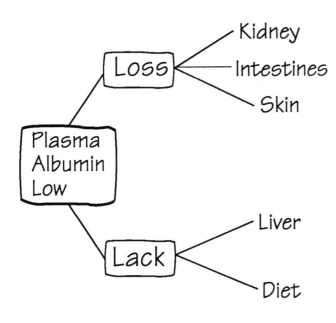

A low plasma albumin in concentration may be due to "loss" or "lack" of total plasma albumin.

Loss can occur through the glomeruli (nephrotic syndrome), or through the gut (protein-losing enteropathy), or through the skin (burns, exudative skin disease).

Lack can occur through failure of manufacture (liver disease), or dietary inadequacy (kwashiorkor; intestinal malabsorption).

Normal Plasma Albumin

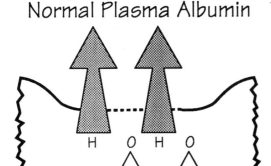

2. Edema With A Normal Plasma Albumin

If the albumin level in the plasma is normal, then the mechanism of the edema is an increased capillary hydrostatic pressure.

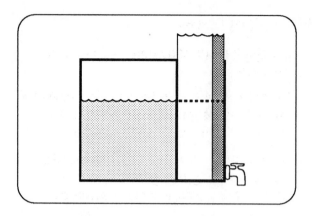

Total plasma and interstitial volume will be increased and the neck veins will be visible indicating a raised venous pressure.

Volume expansion in this instance is therefore distributed throughout the entirety of the E.C.F.

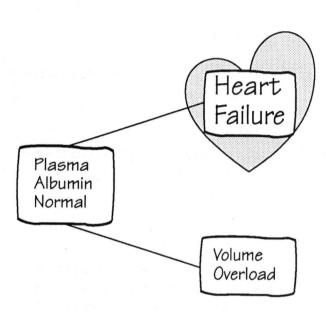

One cause is cardiac failure. Here effective forward flow is reduced, due to a defective pump, and volume accumulates "behind" the heart leading to venous engorgement.

Reduced forward flow means that effective renal blood flow falls. This sets in motion all the mechanisms in the kidney that will retain sodium (and water) and thus continue to increase the edema. The blood pressure is often low because of reduced cardiac output.

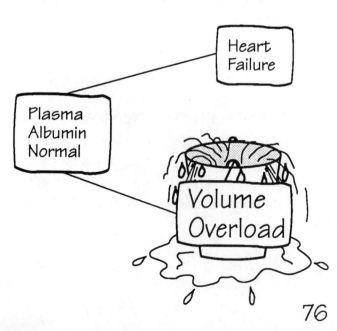

Another cause is volume overload where sodium and water are retained in the presence of a healthy heart. This is usually caused by primary renal disease such as acute glomerulo-nephritis.

It will also be seen in acute or advanced chronic renal failure if sodium loading has been allowed to occur.

In these situations, the venous pressure and the arterial pressure are both increased. Expanded volume in the pulmonary circulation causes breathlessness due to interstitial pulmonary edema.

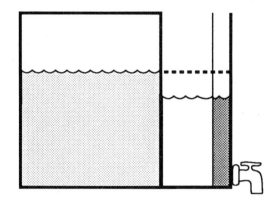

✳ Sodium Loss

The cardinal sign of sodium loss is volume depletion.

The plasma volume will be reduced, resulting in low blood pressure and rapid pulse, more obvious on standing.

The interstitial volume will be diminished as indicated by lack of edema, reduced skin turgor, sunken eyes, and dry mucosal surfaces.

The patient will be thirsty and may also be nauseated.

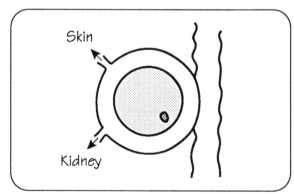

Vomiting ①

E.C.F

I.C.F.

Fistula ③

Diarrhea ②

The common site for sodium (and water) loss is from the intestine due to:

1) Vomiting
2) Diarrhea
3) External fistula, usually the result of some surgical problem.

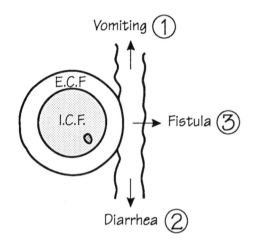

Skin

Kidney

A second site for loss is from the kidney itself in disease that predominantly effects the tubules. Examples include atrophic pyelonephritis and obstructive uropathy.

A third site is from the skin in uncontrolled sweating such as may occur in an extremely hot environment.

Losses from the intestine can, for practical purposes, be considered as losses of E.C.F. volume, and are usually approximately isotonic.

Above the pylorus they are isotonic but with an excess of hydrogen, chloride, and potassium. So the patient with pyloric stenosis will develop

1) Isotonic E.C.F. volume depletion
2) Hypochloremia
3) Alkalosis
4) Hypokalemia

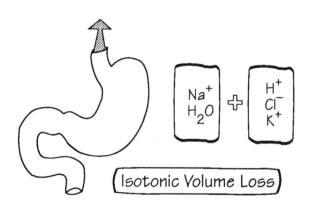

Na^+ H_2O ➕ H^+ Cl^- K^+

Isotonic Volume Loss

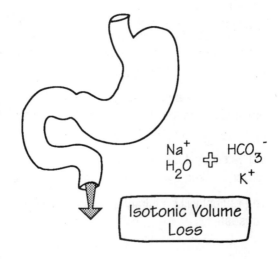

Isotonic Volume Loss

Na^+
H_2O + HCO_3^-
K^+

Losses from below the pylorus including the whole small intestine and proximal colon are also isotonic, but with an excess of bicarbonate and potassium.

The patient with small intestinal diarrhea (e.g. cholera) will therefore develop

1) Isotonic E.C.F. volume depletion
2) Metabolic acidosis
3) Hypokalemia

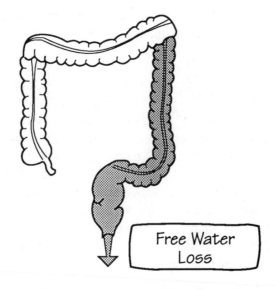

Free Water Loss

Only with diarrhea from the distal part of the large intestine are the losses hypotonic, with losses of water being greater than of solutes.

The Meaning of the Plasma Sodium Concentration

The normal plasma sodium concentration varies between 135 and 145 millimoles per litre. Contrary to what most students expect, the plasma sodium concentration is a poor index of loss or gain of total body sodium.

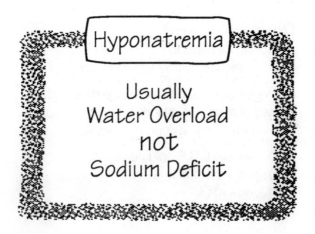

Hyponatremia

Usually Water Overload not Sodium Deficit

Hyponatremia

Since sodium is usually lost in isotonic solution, it is usually recognized by volume depletion and the plasma sodium remains normal.

Hyponatremia is seldom present unless E.C.F. volume losses have been replaced by water, thus producing dilution and hyponatremia.

Hyponatremia is usually a sign of relative water overload, not sodium deficit.

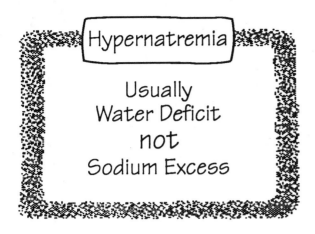

✳ Hypernatremia

Hypernatremia

Hypernatremia is usually a sign of relative water deficit, not sodium overload.

Since these events are largely due to a mismanagement of the handling of water rather than sodium, they will be discussed in more depth in chapter 7.

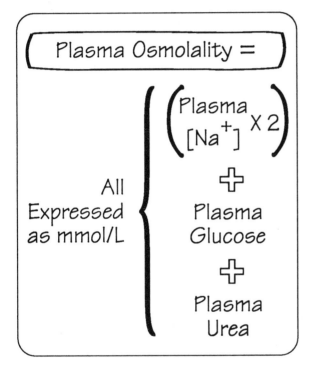

Pseudohyponatremia

The presence of large amounts of an osmotically active solute, not normally present in the E.C.F. will attract extra water into the E.C.F. and dilute the sodium. An example is a diabetic who, in the absence of insulin, cannot transport glucose into the cells. In this setting, glucose contributes significantly to the osmolality of the plasma, which can be calculated by the equation shown here.

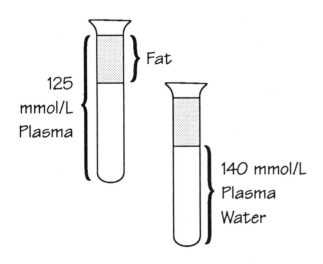

Factitious hyponatremia

Because sodium concentrations are expressed as millimoles per litre of plasma, the plasma sodium concentration may appear to be low if the plasma contains a large volume of substances that replace water.

An example is lipemic plasma that contains large amounts of fat. The sodium concentration may be 125 millimoles per litre of plasma, but is in fact normal when expressed per litre of plasma water.

Chapter 7

The Regulation of Water

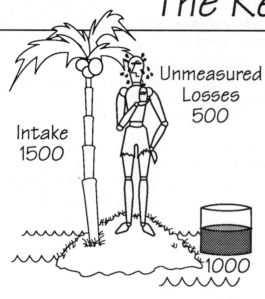

Under normal circumstances we all maintain a water "balance" so that our intake and our losses are equal.

Sources of loss include moistening the expired air, sweating, and of course, the urine.

Because of losses from sites other than the kidney, our urine output is always **less** than our total water intake.

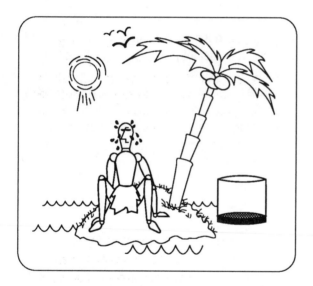

When we are deprived of water, or when our losses by routes other than the urine increase, the urine becomes smaller in volume and more concentrated.

We can all recognize this by the reduction in volume and more intense colour of the urine we pass in hot weather when our losses via perspiration increase.

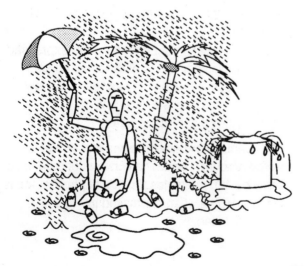

When our fluid intake is high, the weather is cool and our unmeasured losses are small, our urine output will increase and its colour will fade.

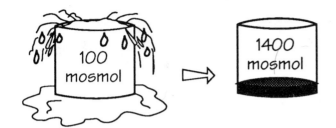

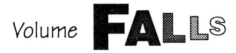

Volume **FALLS**

Concentration **RISES**

The ability to vary the volume and concentration of the urine in accordance with our needs to lose or retain water is an illustration of the precise role of the kidney as a regulator of normal function.

When we have a plentiful supply of water, the urine may be much more dilute than plasma, when water is in short supply it can be as much as four times as concentrated as plasma.

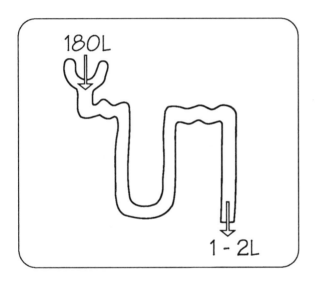

In the previous chapter it was noted that the total volume of glomerular filtrate each day, for an adult, is about 180 litres, but the final urine output is a litre or two, indicating that about 99% of filtered water is reabsorbed.

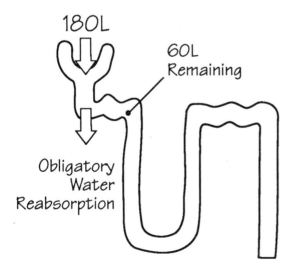

Most of this volume is reabsorbed in the proximal tubule as a passive osmotic event, secondary to the active movement of sodium and chloride out of the lumen. For each 140 millimoles of sodium reabsorbed, one litre of water is bound to follow as an osmotic inevitability.

This water reabsorption is obligatory and will vary to the extent that sodium reabsorption varies. Up to 120 litres may be reabsorbed in this way, but it is all "captive" water, tied to the osmotic effects of active ionic transport.

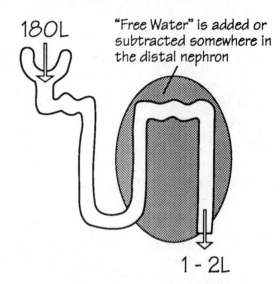

180L

"Free Water" is added or subtracted somewhere in the distal nephron

1 - 2L

Losing or retaining water independently of these osmotic inevitabilities implies the reabsorption or non-reabsorption of water free of such osmotic demands.

Thus the term "free water" has been coined for water that is added to the urine (thus diluting it) or subtracted from the urine (thus concentrating it) without any initial movement of solutes. This all takes place beyond the end of the proximal tubule.

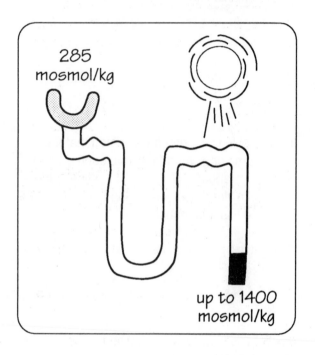

285 mosmol/kg

up to 1400 mosmol/kg

Some Basic Observations

The observations which led to the understanding of this mechanism offer a fascinating glimpse into a piece of physiologic history which began with the observation that whilst the glomerular filtrate is always isotonic with plasma, the urine may be as concentrated as 1200 or even 1400 milliosmoles per kilogram.

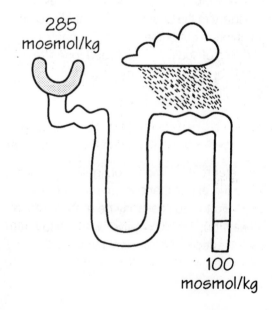

285 mosmol/kg

100 mosmol/kg

On the other hand, the urine may be as dilute as 100 milliosmoles per kilogram or even less which is, of course, much more dilute than plasma.

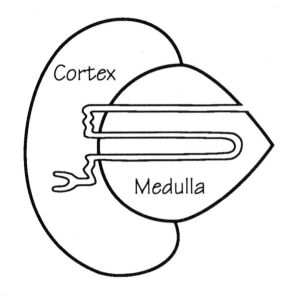

Cortex

Medulla

Along with these facts goes the observation that the configuration of the nephron is highly distinctive, particularly those nephrons arising close to the medulla. Between the proximal and distal tubules of about 30% of nephrons the loop of Henle plunges down deep into the medulla only to return again (like a hairpin loop) to the cortex; then the most distal part of the entire nephron (the collecting duct) runs back through the medulla again, parallel to the loops of Henle.

For years anatomists and physiologists wondered why the nephron was constructed in this way and the discovery of the link between structure and function was an exciting story.

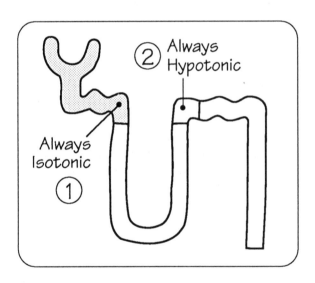

② Always Hypotonic

Always Isotonic ①

Two important facts were found in animals by micropuncture. These were:

1) That the filtered urine remained isotonic with plasma up to the end of the proximal tubule, whatever the final urine concentration.

2) That the urine was always hypotonic at the end of the loop of Henle, whatever the final urine concentration.

Clearly, something was happening in the loop of Henle to dilute the urine.

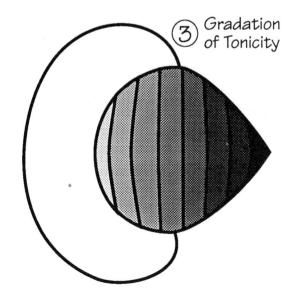

③ Gradation of Tonicity

A third observation was that the tonicity of the tissues in the medulla showed a gradation, being concentrated at the tip and isotonic at the corticomedullary junction.

In studies of a wide range of mammals, this gradient was most marked in those which were able to concentrate their urine most impressively.

It was also noted that the longer the medullary papilla and the longer the loops of Henle, the greater was the ability to concentrate the final urine (for example in desert rodents).

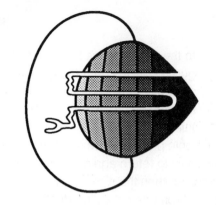

Against this background it seemed clear that the anatomical arrangement of the tubule was related in more than a casual way to the osmotic gradients within the medulla, but its relationship to the way in which the kidney regulated water balance was still not clear.

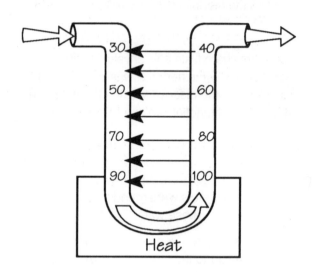

Heat

A Countercurrent System

Some investigators, however, recognized that this arrangement looked as if it might function like a "countercurrent" exchange system familiar to engineers.

In a heat exchange system, for example, heat can be conserved by placing the incoming cold water close to the outgoing hot water, thus trapping heat that would otherwise be wasted. This same general principle was in fact found to be applicable to the urinary concentrating mechanism.

It was then shown that the ascending limb of the loop of Henle had special properties.

1) The wall of the entire ascending limb allows solutes to move out of the lumen but does not allow water to follow the osmotic gradient this creates. In effect it is waterproof.

2) The thick ascending limb is the site of a transport system (powered by the Na^+/K^+ ATP-ase at its basolateral surface) which utilizes a Na^+, K^+, 2 Cl^- transporter (see page 68) where Cl^- is the rate-limiting factor.

3) Whilst the thin ascending limb does not have an active transport system, it is relatively permeable to NaCl. The osmotic environment that develops outside the tubule favours diffusion of NaCl out of the ascending limb with the result that the entire ascending limb can be regarded as behaving uniformly even though only part of it has an active pump.

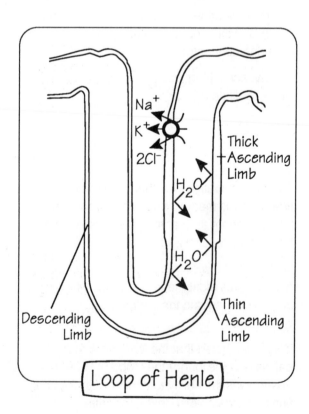

Loop of Henle

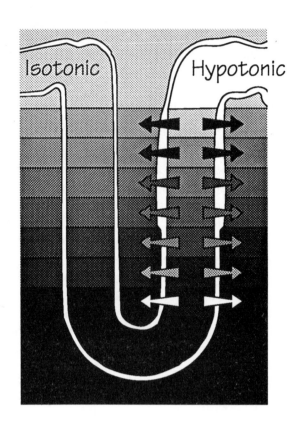

A Countercurrent Multiplier

As a result of these processes, and as fluid moves slowly through the loop of Henle, each step of the way up the ascending limb, solute is removed from the tubule and added to the interstitium, leaving water behind.

As this process is repeated over and over again in many small steps, it can be seen that the urine becomes progressively more dilute. At any given level, the interstitial fluid is relatively more concentrated than the urine in the ascending limb. Thus, by the end of the loop of Henle the urine has become hypotonic.

As a result of small concentration steps, multiplied many times over, a gradient of solute concentration is built up throughout the medulla with the greatest concentration at its tip.

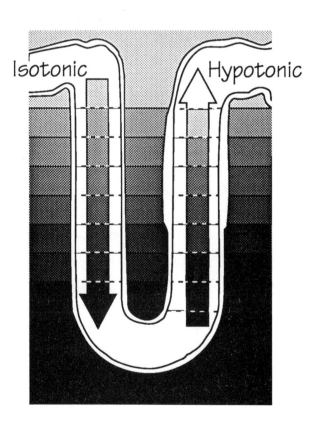

Because the descending limb of the loop of Henle is freely permeable to water it will share all of the concentration steps of the interstitium around it. Water moves passively across its wall to equalize osmolalities.

This process of concentration of the interstitium and dilution in the ascending limb of the tubule by a series of very tiny steps will go on until an equilibrium is reached. This will depend upon the rate of flow of the urine, the length of the loop, and presumably the number of pump sites. The "hairpin" configuration of the loop is, of course, essential in order to "trap" and maintain the concentration gradient.

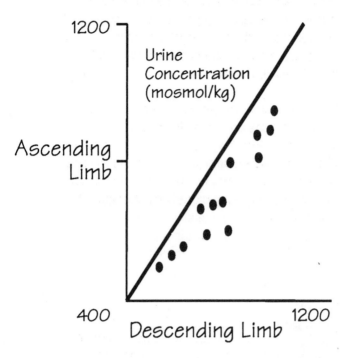

1200

Urine
Concentration
(mosmol/kg)

Ascending
Limb

400   1200
Descending Limb

After Jamison etal Am. J. Physiol 212 357 (1967)

Support for this theory has been shown by a number of experiments such as the one shown here. As the theory predicted, micropuncture studies in animals showed that at all levels of the loop of Henle, the fluid in the ascending limb was always less concentrated than the fluid in the descending limb.

Recent studies have added more refinement to our understanding of the way in which this system functions. For example, in the presence of ADH water moves out of the cortical collecting tubules raising the concentration of urea in the tubule which is relatively impermeable to urea at this site. But when the fluid enters the medullary collecting duct, this relative impermeability disappears and urea moves out of the interstitium to contribute to the hypertonicity there. In fact, the urea gets trapped by the counter current system and contributes almost half of the osmolar gradient in the medulla.

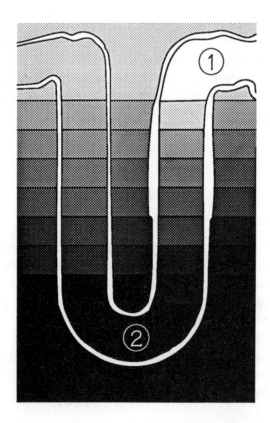

The whole system is more complex than has been outlined here but this forms a reasonable basis for understanding the concepts involved.

So far it is clear that, at all times, the properties of the loop of Henle will result in:

1) A dilute urine at the end of the ascending limb, and

2) A concentrated urine at the tip of the hairpin in the medulla.

The mechanism of urinary *dilution* has therefore been explained, but how do we now explain urinary concentration by the end of the collecting tubule?

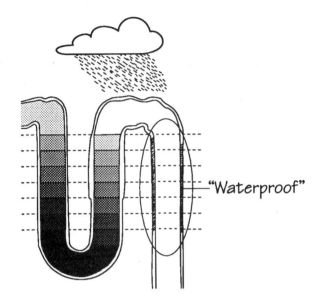

"Waterproof"

Another anatomical fact now becomes very important. The collecting duct plunges down through the medulla amongst the loops of Henle and through the concentration gradient of the medullary interstitium.

Under conditions where water conservation is not needed, the urine remains dilute until it leaves the kidney because the collecting duct is effectively "waterproof" just as is the ascending limb of the loop of Henle. Thus, the urine is not affected by the osmotic gradients through which it passes.

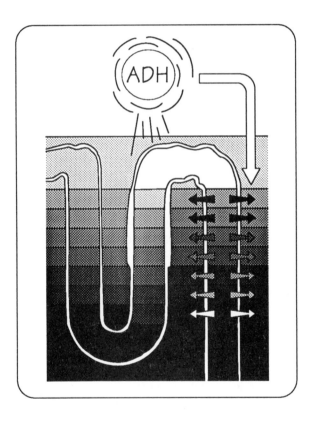

ADH

When, however, water conservation is required, anti-diuretic hormone (ADH) released from the hypothalamus, renders the wall of the collecting duct permeable to water. As a result, the osmotic effects of the interstitium cause the removal of water from the collecting duct, thus concentrating the final urine.

As well as rendering the collecting ducts permeable to water, ADH may also increase the activity of the pump in the ascending limb of the loop of Henle. This will also favour distal water recovery by increasing the osmotic gradients but has not been proven to occur in man.

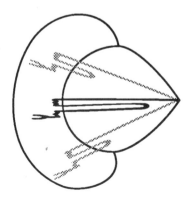

Two final notes must be made.

The first is that in man, only perhaps 30% of nephrons have long loops of Henle and it is only these that are responsible for setting up the conditions whereby medullary gradients become established and urine concentration may occur. The loss of these nephrons (by disease of the medulla, for example) will upset the concentrating ability of the kidney as a whole.

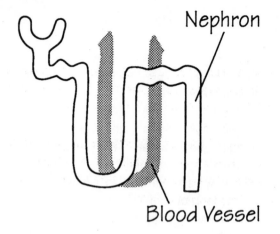

Nephron

Blood Vessel

A Countercurrent Exchanger

The second point is that the blood vessels coursing through the medulla also have a "hairpin" configuration. This is essential to maintain the concentration gradients set up by the countercurrent multiplier of the loop of Henle.

The loops of the blood vessels act as a **countercurrent exchanger** and maintain the gradients rather than washing them out as would occur if they went straight through the medulla.

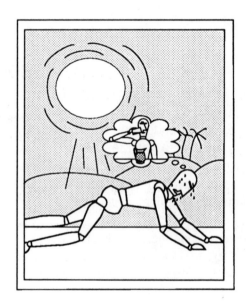

Clinical Examples of Disordered Water Handling

1. Water Depletion

The cardinal symptom of water depletion is thirst.

The laboratory companion of thirst is a high plasma sodium which indicates a high E.C.F. osmolality.

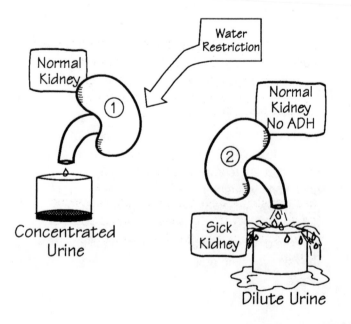

Normal Kidney

Water Restriction

Normal Kidney No ADH

①

②

Concentrated Urine

Sick Kidney

Dilute Urine

The response to water depletion can be classified in the following ways.

1) If the depletion is due to water restriction with normal kidneys, the urine will be highly concentrated, and the patient will be passing small amounts of urine.

2) If however, it is due to loss of water from the kidney in the absence of any restriction of water intake, the urine will be dilute and the patient will be passing large amounts of urine. Such losses may occur as a result of renal disease or as a result of some abnormality of ADH production or its effect.

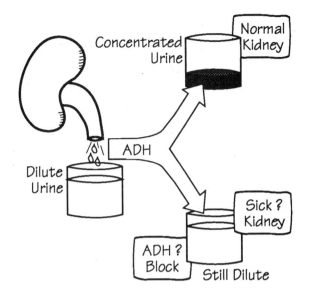

If such renal water loss can be corrected by the administration of ADH then it is due to a defect in ADH production with a normal kidney.

If the defect cannot be corrected by ADH then it must be due either to an abnormal kidney that cannot respond to ADH or to some block to the peripheral action of ADH.

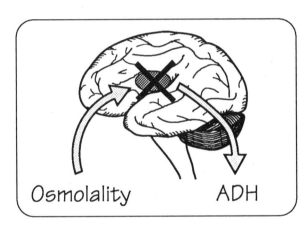

ADH RELATED WATER DEPLETION

If the defect can be corrected by ADH administration, then it implies a healthy kidney but some defect in the production or release of ADH from the hypothalamus.

This condition is characterized by profound polyuria and thirst and is called diabetes insipidus. It has already been referred to in Chapter 5.

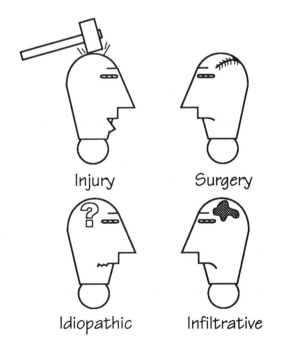

It may be caused by trauma, with fracture of the base of the skull, complications of cranial surgery (particularly pituitary gland surgery), or by infiltrative processes such as basal meningitis or neoplasm.

Many cases, however, appear with no obvious cause and have to be classified as "idiopathic" which simply means that the cause is not known.

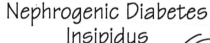

Medullary Disease

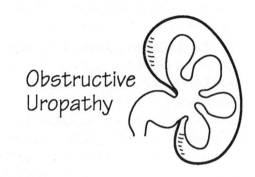

Obstructive
Uropathy

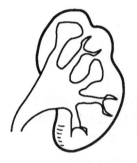

Atrophic
Pyelonephritis

Nephrogenic Diabetes
Insipidus

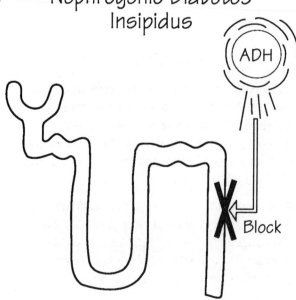

ADH

Block

ADH INDEPENDENT WATER LOSS

There are three mechanisms by which disordered kidney function may lead to water depletion which is unrelated to ADH production.

1) ABNORMAL KIDNEY FUNCTION

One is by structural damage to the medulla of the kidney involving the long loops of Henle which are responsible for generating concentration gradients in the medulla. Selective loss of these nephrons can cause a selective loss of concentrating ability without major disturbance of overall glomerular function.

Damage to tubular function in such situations is seldom limited only to "free water" reabsorption and such patients usually have solute dependent loss of water as well. Examples are atrophic pyelonephritis and obstructive uropathy.

2) BLOCKADE OF ADH ACTION

The second mechanism is of renal non-response to ADH due to a functional abnormality of the tubule. This is referred to as "nephrogenic diabetes insipidus".

This condition may be a spontaneously occurring problem in a male infant whose immature kidney fails to respond to normal ADH.

It may, however, be a side effect of certain drugs, particularly lithium carbonate which is widely used in manic- depressive illness. Lithium appears to block the tubular actions of ADH.

Cortical Disease

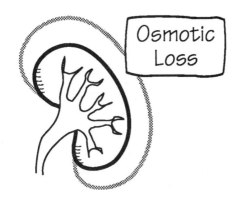

Osmotic
Loss

Chronic
Glomerulonephritis

Diabetes Mellitus

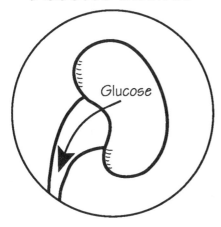

Glucose

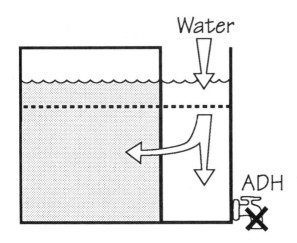

Water

ADH

3) CORTICAL DISEASE

Another mechanism of ADH block is an osmotic effect due to high levels of filtered solutes in the relatively few remaining nephrons that are functioning in advancing cortical disease such as chronic glomerulonephritis.

Those nephrons that still survive are handling a much higher load of solutes, such as urea, than they were when all nephrons were functioning. Such solutes provide an osmotic load which will increase tubular flow and "wash out" the medullary concentration gradient. As a result ADH can no longer be effective. This explains the polyuria of most patients with chronic renal failure.

A similar mechanism operates in uncontrolled diabetes mellitus where glucose is the osmotic solute in an otherwise normal kidney.

Because of the high blood sugar and the consequent "overflow" into the glomerular filtrate, the ability of the tubule to reabsorb glucose is overwhelmed. Glucose is left within the tubule and provides an effective osmotic load which washes out the concentration gradient and prevents ADH being effective.

2. Water Retention

Water retention occurs whenever water intake exceeds the ability of the body to excrete an excess load. Since a water load is evenly distributed throughout body water, it will cause proportionately similar expansion of E.C.F. and I.C.F. compartments.

It will also dilute the solute concentrations in the body fluids. Hyponatremia is therefore an invariable finding which indicates an excess of water and not a deficit of sodium. ADH production will normally be shut off by such events.

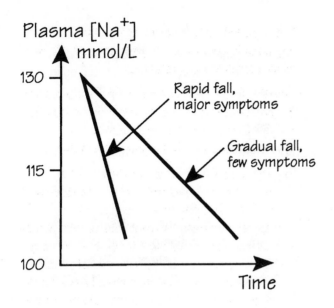

Retention of large volumes of water over a short period of time causes a rapid fall in serum sodium and the development of major neurological symptoms due to osmotic shifts of water into the I.C.F., most notable in the intracranial structures.

Gradual retention of water is, however, a more common clinical situation and does not produce dramatic cerebral signs. A gradual fall in plasma sodium with the gradual development of headache and confusion may occur but, when slowly developing, a plasma sodium as low as 100 millimoles per litre may be surprisingly asymptomatic.

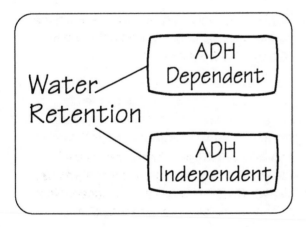

There are two major mechanisms whereby water is retained.

1) Due to the effects of ADH acting upon the kidney.

2) Due to failure of an abnormal kidney to excrete a water load, regardless of ADH activity.

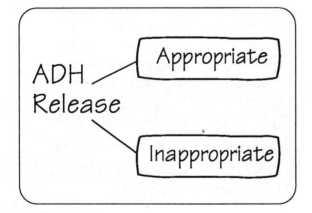

ADH DEPENDENT WATER RETENTION

ADH dependent water retention may be divided into two categories.

1) Those which depend upon known physiologic stimuli and are therefore "appropriate".

2) Those unrelated to any normal mechanism for ADH release and therefore "inappropriate".

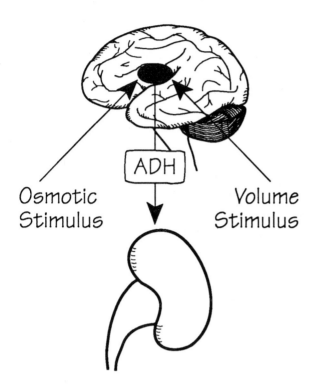

Osmotic
Stimulus

Volume
Stimulus

It is important at this stage to note that in the physiologic control of body water there are two major stimuli to ADH release.

1) The first is the stimulus of changing plasma osmolality which leads to changing output of ADH in response to stimulation of osmoreceptors in the hypothalamus.

2) The second is a stimulus resulting from persistent hypovolemia. ADH released by this stimulus can over-ride "osmotic appropriateness" so that volume stimuli may continue to cause the release of ADH long after the plasma osmolality has fallen to a point where ADH release would have been expected to be cut off. Such volume stimuli may relate as much to volume maldistribution as to overall fluid volume loss.

Whatever the nature of the stimulus, the result will be the retention of "free water" without accompanying solutes.

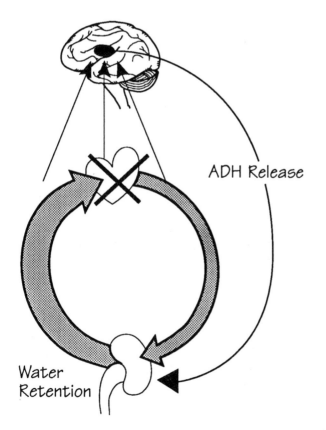

ADH Release

Water
Retention

This is seen in heart failure where all the sodium-retaining mechanisms are in play, but still the effective forward flow is inadequate in spite of the presence of obvious edema.

In such situations afferent stimuli reach the hypothalamus from a number of receptors which monitor "volume" in some way and probably include sites in the aortic arch, the right and left side of the heart and the great veins.

The resulting ADH release causes water retention (and hyponatremia) in patients who are often already being treated with potent diuretics and considered to have become "resistant" to them.

Because it has a physiologic explanation such ADH production is "appropriate".

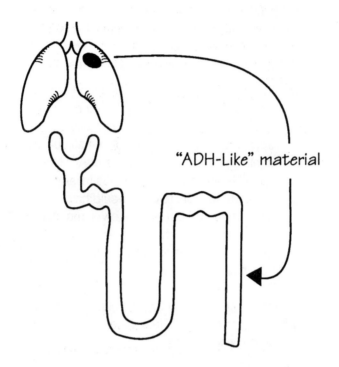

Sometimes, however, water is retained due to ADH release which has no physiologic explanation. ADH (or ADH-like material) is being produced independent of any osmotic or volume stimulus.

ADH-like material may be produced by a neoplasm, most commonly a carcinoma of the lung. This results in the syndrome of "inappropriate ADH secretion" (SIADH).

The same situation can occur when true ADH activity is enhanced by the action of a drug (e.g. chlopropamide) which either causes increased release of ADH from the hypothalamus or an increased effect of ADH on the kidney.

"ADH-Like" material

The laboratory indicators of this situation are a low plasma sodium with an inappropriately concentrated urine. Because free water retention causes expansion of all body compartments including the E.C.F., the kidney tends to release sodium into the urine since the volume expansion inhibits sodium retaining mechanisms. Thus, edema does not occur and volume expansion is not clinically obvious.

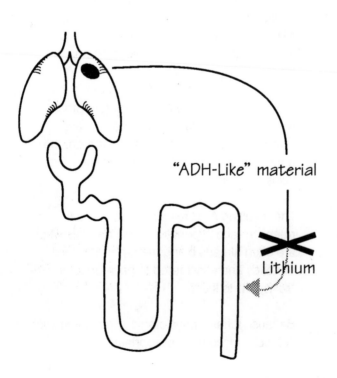

"ADH-Like" material

Lithium

This syndrome can be treated by restriction of water intake or by attempting to block the action of ADH on the renal collecting ducts with drugs such as lithium carbonate or demeclocycline.

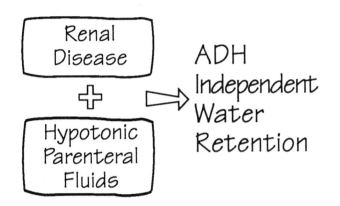

ADH INDEPENDENT WATER RETENTION

Water retention independent of ADH is due to renal disease which limits the excretion of a water load. Since such patients become both volume expanded and diluted, they are seldom thirsty and continued water retention is usually secondary to some non-physiologic route of fluid intake (usually intravenous infusion).

This is therefore mainly an iatrogenic problem occurring in hospitalized patients.

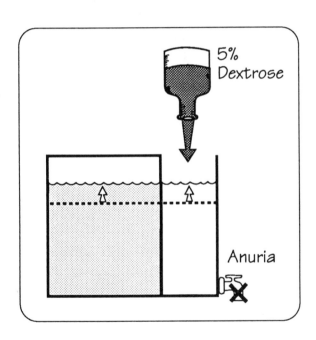

An example of such a situation arises when a patient receives continued loading with intravenous dextrose and water after oliguria has developed.

In the early phase of acute oliguric renal failure the inability to excrete a water load may be unnoticed at a time when fluid intake is being encouraged.

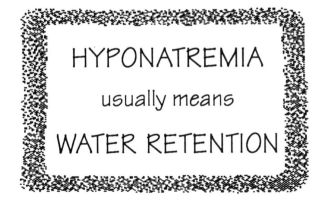

Retention of "free water" in all these situations will cause hyponatremia, and as mentioned in Chapter 6, a low serum sodium is usually due to water retention and not due to sodium loss.

Chapter 8

The Regulation of Hydrogen Ions

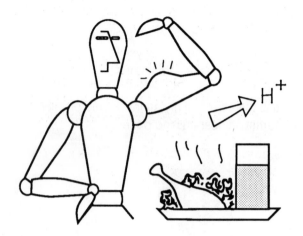

On a normal North American protein-rich diet and with normal metabolic activity, the body is constantly producing protons which threaten the stability of the hydrogen ion concentration upon which the cells rely if they are to function normally. In health most are removed by oxidation. If not, they have to be dealt with in other ways, which is the topic of the present chapter.

Some basic definitions relating to hydrogen ions have been given on pages 23 and 24.

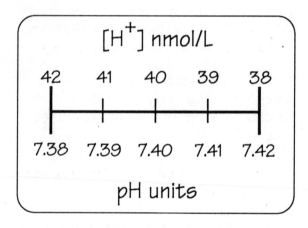

Remember that a proton is a hydrogen atom that has given up an electron and is the same as a hydrogen ion.

An acid is any substance that can give up a proton, whilst a base can receive a proton.

Normal E.C.F. hydrogen ion concentration is about 40 nanomoles per litre (40×10^{-9} moles per litre) which is a pH of 7.4. In the events of everyday life the variation of extracellular pH is very narrow. Around this normal range one nanomole of hydrogen ions per litre equates with 0.01 pH unit (a convenient coincidence).

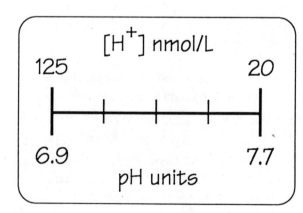

In abnormal situations, much wider ranges may be seen, and this diagram indicates the kind of maximal aberrations beyond which the limits of survival are usually passed. In practice a pH of 6.9 or 7.7 will only be seen in profound pathological situations.

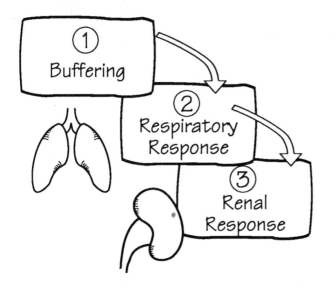

Three mechanisms are available to regulate changes in the pH of the E.C.F. and they operate in the sequence shown here.

Buffering is more or less immediate, the respiratory response is delayed and the renal response is the slowest to develop.

Buffering traps free hydrogen ions without disposing of them. Since they are generated in an uneven manner, buffering is essential to the maintenance of a stable pH whilst evening out the delivery of free hydrogen ions to a system which will finally dispose of them. This system includes the lungs and the kidneys.

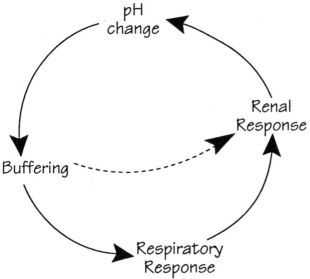

In physiological situations where large and rapid changes of pH are not allowed to occur, a smooth coordination of these three regulating steps provides a precise and continuous control of the pH of the E.C.F. thus keeping it within the narrow limits indicated on the previous page.

Buffering

The concept of "buffering" is well illustrated by this old experiment.

If hydrochloric acid is added to a bucket of water, the pH drops rapidly. If the same amount of hydrochloric acid is infused into a dog with the same total body water as the bucket, little fall in pH occurs. The hydrogen ion load has been "buffered".

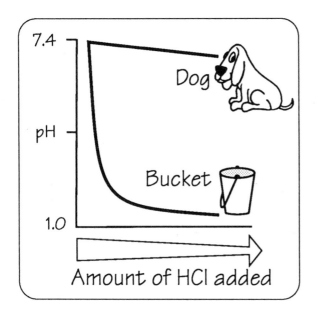

Buffering is achieved by the binding of hydrogen ions in weak acids. Because they do not completely dissociate, they limit the amount of free hydrogen ion available and act like a sponge which soaks up hydrogen ions.

Strong Acid

$$HCl \rightleftharpoons H^+ + Cl^-$$

Hydrochloric acid is a strong acid and almost completely dissociates to produce a high concentration of hydrogen ions.

Weak Acid

$$H_2PO_4^- \rightleftharpoons H^+ + HPO_4^{2-}$$

Dihydrogen phosphate on the other hand is a weak acid and only partially dissociates to give less free hydrogen ions then an equimolar amount of hydrochloric acid. It can therefore act as a buffer.

① $$H^+ \equiv K_A \frac{[H^+ \, donor]}{[H^+ \, acceptor]}$$

can be re-written as:

② $$pH \equiv pK_A + log \frac{[H^+ \, acceptor]}{[H^+ \, donor]}$$

The Buffer Equation

The relationship between the two sides of a "buffer reaction" can be expressed by the general equation of Henderson (1) which is based on the law of mass action where K_A is the dissociation constant for the acid in question.

However, the use of actual hydrogen ion concentration has not gained general clinical acceptance and so "Henderson's equation" has been modified, by a simple mathematical trick, to express hydrogen ion concentration as pH. In this form it carries the names of Henderson and Hasselbalch (2).

The two equations say the same thing but in different ways and to avoid confusion we will stay with pH as the unit of hydrogen ion concentration.

① $$NH_3 + H^+ \rightleftharpoons NH_4^+$$
pK 9.2

② $$HPO_4^{2-} + H^+ \rightleftharpoons H_2PO_4^-$$
pK 6.8

③ $$HCO_3^- + H^+ \rightleftharpoons H_2CO_3$$
pK 6.1

Buffer Reactions

The pK_A for any buffer is a constant which depends upon the buffer being considered. It is the pH at which the reaction is evenly balanced between the two components of a buffer pair so that each is present in equal concentration.

$$pH = 6.8 + \log \frac{[HPO_4^{2-}]}{H_2PO_4^{-}}$$

For phosphate, as an example, the reaction can be represented as shown here. In any buffer reaction the relationship between pH and the "buffer pair" represented on each side of the reaction is mathematically predictable. If the pH is known, then the ionic concentrations of the reactants can be calculated.

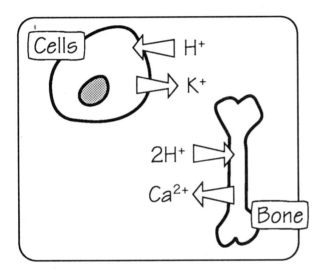

Intracellular Buffers

In the body as a whole, 60% or more of buffering occurs inside the cells. To enter the cells, the hydrogen ions exchange with potassium ions, which explains why a sudden acid load may be associated with an increase in the potassium concentration in the E.C.F.

In states of long-standing systemic acidosis hydrogen ions may enter bony tissue in exchange for calcium ions and this can eventually lead to demineralisation of the bone (osteomalacia).

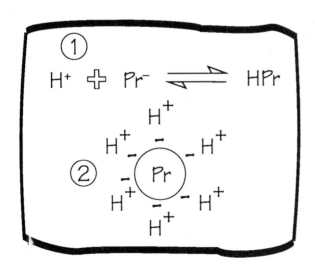

The most important intracellular buffers are proteins and include hemoglobin in the red cells.

The buffer equation for a protein is shown here (1) but in fact most proteins function as polyanions with a number of sites where cations may bind (2).

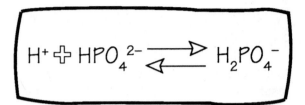

$$H^+ + HPO_4^{2-} \rightleftharpoons H_2PO_4^-$$

Extracellular Buffers

Extracellular buffers such as phosphate only have a limited capacity to soak up hydrogen ions. They rapidly become saturated as the end product accumulates and brings the reaction to equilibrium and at this point have no further capacity to buffer hydrogen ions.

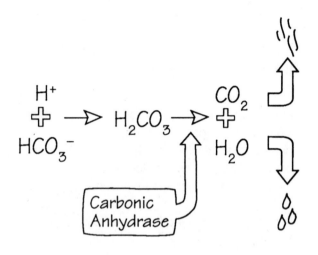

$$H^+ + HCO_3^- \rightarrow H_2CO_3 \rightarrow CO_2 + H_2O$$

Carbonic Anhydrase

However, the reaction which converts bicarbonate to carbonic acid does not become saturated, and for this reason, the value of bicarbonate as a buffer in the E.C.F. is unique.

The end products of the reaction can be dissipated: Carbon dioxide via the lungs and water into the general water pool in the body.

The presence of the enzyme carbonic anhydrase accelerates the otherwise fairly slow reaction that releases CO_2 and H_2O from carbonic acid.

$$pH \equiv 6.1 + \log \frac{[HCO_3^-]}{H_2CO_3}$$

The relationship between pH and the action of bicarbonate as a buffer can be mathematically predicted by the Henderson-Hasselbalch equation. Clearly if any two of the variables are known the third can be calculated, and many nomograms exist whereby such calculations are rendered simple.

OR

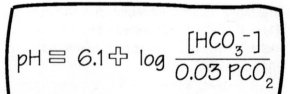

$$pH \equiv 6.1 + \log \frac{[HCO_3^-]}{0.03\ PCO_2}$$

The equation can be rewritten in a number of ways which accept the fact that carbonic acid is in equilibrium with the dissolved carbon dioxide in the body fluids. Carbon dioxide is expressed in terms of its partial pressure, using the term Pco_2.

In conceptual form, which simplifies things yet further, the relationship can be rewritten in this way, which will prove useful in the clinical situations to be discussed later.

It is important to recognize that this relationship means that the pH will vary as the bicarbonate and PCO_2 change. In other words, if other things remain constant:

1) Removing bicarbonate, raising the PCO_2 or adding free hydrogen ions will all have the same effect - a fall of pH.

2) Adding bicarbonate, lowering PCO_2 or removing free hydrogen ions will all produce the same effect - a rise of pH.

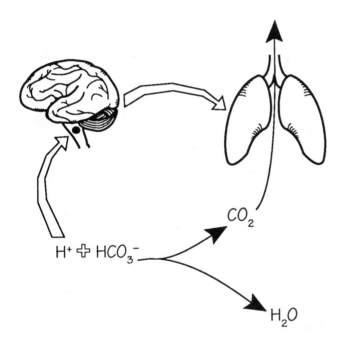

$$pH \quad \text{depends upon} \quad \frac{[HCO_3^-]}{PCO_2}$$

The Respiratory Response

It is now apparent what constitutes the respiratory response. In effect, hydrogen ions can be turned into water with carbon dioxide as a by-product. The reaction can keep moving from left to right, without any saturation due to buildup of end products of the reaction, because carbon dioxide can be rapidly excreted through the lungs.

The stimulus to increased ventilation is probably an increase of hydrogen ion concentration sensed by cells in the brain stem. Provided the lungs are healthy, they can increase ventilation to excrete a large amount of carbon dioxide.

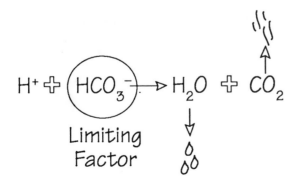

$$H^+ + \boxed{HCO_3^-} \rightarrow H_2O + CO_2$$

Limiting Factor

The limit to this reaction in the presence of normal lungs is therefore not a buildup of the end products of the reaction (water or carbon dioxide) but a "running down" of available bicarbonate to fuel the continued buffering of hydrogen ion.

The Kidney makes HCO_3^-

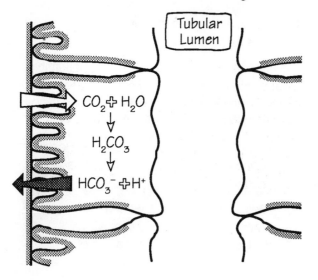

The Renal Response

This is where the renal response comes in. The kidney has the capability of regenerating the bicarbonate supply and in effect does this by reversing the chemical process involved in the respiratory response.

Carbon dioxide diffuses into the cells of the renal tubule and leads to the production of bicarbonate which returns to the E.C.F. to replenish the E.C.F. bicarbonate.

and as a result:
The Kidney must excrete H^+

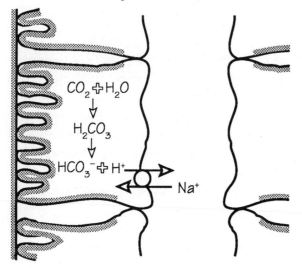

The beauty of this mechanism is that for every bicarbonate ion that is returned to the E.C.F. one hydrogen ion is ejected into the tubular lumen, thus providing an additional mechanism for removing hydrogen ion from the E.C.F.

Hydrogen ion moves out of the cell in exchange for sodium through the Na^+/H^+ antiporter in the luminal membrane and this process accounts for the majority of hydrogen ions transported into the tubule.

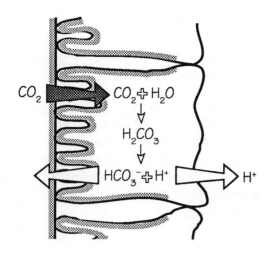

Bicarbonate production, and thus hydrogen ion excretion, will be increased by a rising partial pressure of carbon dioxide which drives the reaction between carbon dioxide and water to produce carbonic acid and then on to bicarbonate and hydrogen ion. This occurs in respiratory failure where the renal response is to excrete hydrogen ions and regenerate bicarbonate to stabilize the pH.

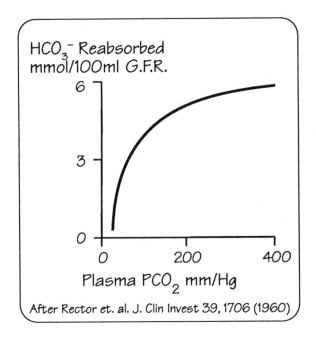

After Rector et. al. J. Clin Invest 39, 1706 (1960)

Some evidence for this is shown by experimental data demonstrating the dramatic effects of plasma P_{CO_2} upon renal bicarbonate generation. This effect is especially marked around the P_{CO_2} levels seen clinically (between 40 and 100 millimeters Hg).

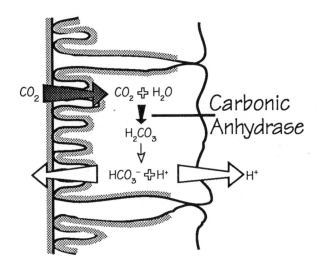

The formation of carbonic acid from water and carbon dioxide is catalyzed by the enzyme carbonic anhydrase.

The presence of this enzyme in the tubular cells favours both this reaction and its continuance to produce bicarbonate and further eliminate hydrogen ions, by continuing to drive the reaction of carbon dioxide and water towards completion.

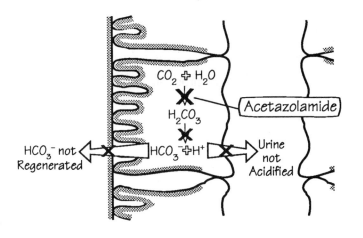

Blocking carbonic anhydrase, with a drug such as acetazolamide, will rapidly block both bicarbonate regeneration and hydrogen ion production by the renal tubule. As a result, filtered bicarbonate will escape in the urine and the buffering capacity in the plasma will fall as the bicarbonate falls. In short, the urine becomes alkaline and the plasma pH falls, a condition called "renal tubular acidosis".

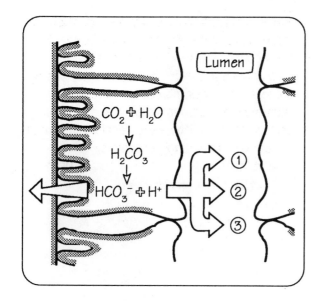

The Disposal of Renal Tubular Hydrogen Ions

It is important at this point, to reiterate that the renal role in pH regulation is to replenish HCO_3^- stores.

Generating HCO_3^- in the tubular cells cannot be done without the coincident production of H^+. This is the "price the kidney must pay" for making new HCO_3^-. Payment of this price requires the existence of a "disposal system" for H^+. Such a system is highly developed in the renal tubule.

Once the hydrogen ion has been secreted into the tubule, it is handled in a way which prevents a fall of pH in the lumen which would otherwise stop further hydrogen ion secretion, since in the proximal tubule the cells cannot transfer hydrogen ions into the lumen against a concentration gradient. There are three ways in which tubular hydrogen ion is handled.
1) Bicarbonate trapping
2) Ammonia production
3) Titratable acid production

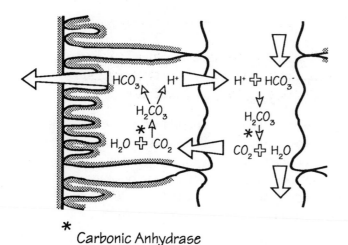

* Carbonic Anhydrase

1. BICARBONATE TRAPPING

The first mechanism occurs when secreted hydrogen ions meet filtered bicarbonate and are trapped in the familiar carbonic acid buffer system. The result is the formation of water and the generation of carbon dioxide which can diffuse back into the tubular cell where it will favour the generation of more bicarbonate and more hydrogen ions. In the proximal tubule carbonic anhydrase is present in the brush border of the luminal membrane and favours this reaction.

In effect, for every bicarbonate ion that is trapped by a hydrogen ion, another bicarbonate ion is generated by the tubular cell. Whilst bicarbonate ions are not reabsorbed as such, the end result is as if every secreted hydrogen ion resulted in the reabsorption of one bicarbonate ion.

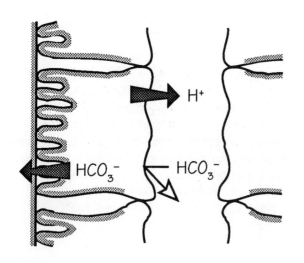

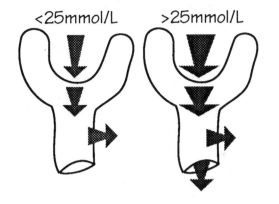

Below a plasma bicarbonate level of about 25 millimoles per litre all filtered bicarbonate is trapped in this way. Above this "threshold" level, bicarbonate may "escape" and appear in the final urine, but in these circumstances bicarbonate excretion, rather than its conservation, will serve the best interests of pH regulation for the whole organism.

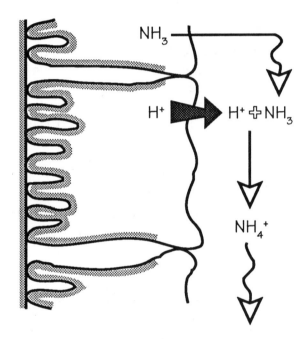

2. AMMONIA PRODUCTION

The second mechanism for handling renal tubular hydrogen ions is by the production of ammonia by the renal tubular cells.

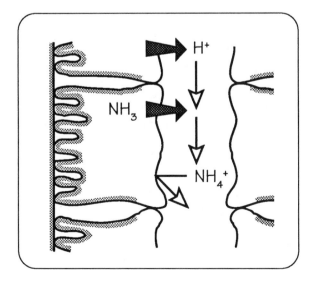

Ammonia is a highly diffusible substance. As soon as it is produced it diffuses rapidly and completely into the tubular lumen. There it meets secreted hydrogen ions and promptly traps them to form ammonium ions. Unlike non-ionic ammonia, ammonium ions cannot diffuse back into the cell, and so stay in the lumen.

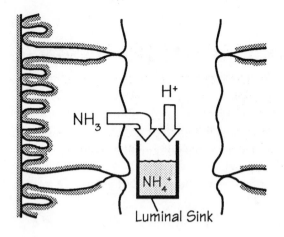

Luminal Sink

So long as ammonia is trapped by hydrogen ions, there will be a gradient for diffusion of ammonia from the cell into the "sink" created by its conversion to non-diffusible ammonium ions.

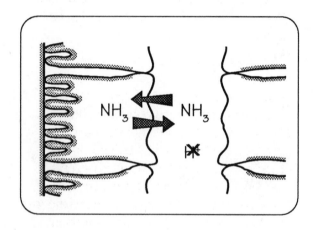

If free hydrogen ions are not present, then the luminal ammonia level will rise and the gradient will disappear. Ammonia will therefore stay within the cells and accumulate, a process which promptly results in a shut-down of further ammonia production. Ammonia is continuously produced only when free hydrogen ions are being produced by the tubule. This means that ammonia production is closely related to the amount of hydrogen ions being produced. Thus the role of this system becomes more important as the need to excrete hydrogen ions and regenerate bicarbonate becomes more persistent.

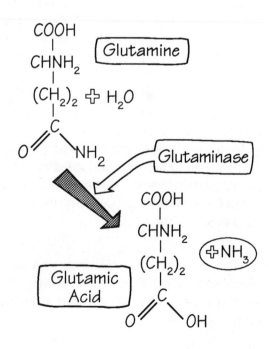

Ammonia production within the tubular cells involves a number of chemical steps which lead to the release of amino groups and to the formation of free ammonia. A final step in that process is shown here.

106

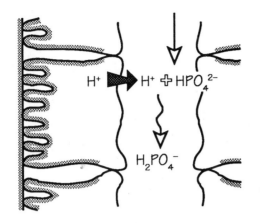

$$H^+ \rightarrow H^+ + HPO_4^{2-}$$

$$H_2PO_4^-$$

3. TITRATABLE ACID PRODUCTION

The third mechanism for managing tubular hydrogen ions is trapping them within buffers (filtered at the glomerulus) other than bicarbonate. The best known example is phosphate which is quantitatively the most important urinary buffer.

Under normal conditions with a urine pH around 6.5, most of the buffering power resides in the phosphate ion and can be measured by back titration to pH 7.4. This is known as titratable acidity.

In the distal parts of the tubule, however, hydrogen ions begin to be pumped out against an increasing concentration gradient. The pH slips downward and the phosphate buffer becomes saturated, so other substances become more important as buffers. In this experiment creatinine is shown to become a more effective buffer as urine pH falls below 5.0, at which point phosphate is becoming less effective. Phosphate is the most important urinary buffer, but not the only one, and of course, titratable acid can only be accommodated by the amount of buffer available to trap it. This means that there is an upper limit to the titratable acidity depending upon the amount of buffer in the glomerular filtrate.

Titratable Acid (%)

100 — Phosphate

Creatinine

0

4 — 7

Urine pH

After Wrong and Davies, Quart J. Med. 28,259 (1959)

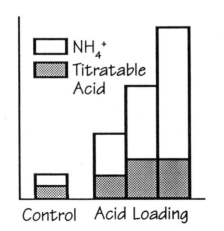

NH₄⁺
Titratable Acid

Control   Acid Loading

When titratable acidity and ammonium formation are compared, as shown here, it is clear that during a control period more than 50% of the hydrogen ions excreted are handled by buffers as titratable acid, whilst less is trapped as ammonium ions.

But when a continuing acid load is provided, ammonium excretion can rise progressively whilst titratable acidity can increase only to the extent that there are suitable buffers available in the glomerular filtrate.

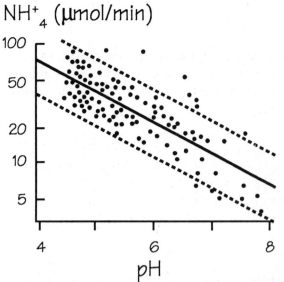

NH$^+_4$ (μmol/min)

After Wrong and Davies, Quart J. Med. 28,259 (1959)

The experimental data shown here illustrate the importance of urinary ammonium. They re-emphasize the fact that the more acidic the urine (and the more saturated titratable acid becomes) the more ammonium is produced.

One final point about these renal mechanisms: Although hydrogen ion is secreted (and bicarbonate regenerated), all along the tubule it is only distally that a significant pH gradient develops. Proximally, H$^+$, transported into the tubular lumen by the Na$^+$/H$^+$ antiporter are so completely trapped that no pH gradient exists even though a large H$^+$ load is handled.

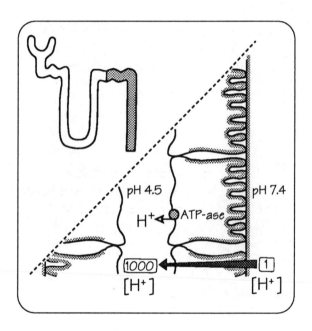

At the end of the distal nephron, however, H$^+$ can be transported against a steep gradient as urinary buffers become successively saturated. This is achieved by an ATP-ase dependent H$^+$ pump in the luminal membrane of the intercalated cells which comprise about one third of the cells in the cortical collecting duct and a higher proportion of cells in the outer medullary collecting duct.

The final urine pH in man can approach 4.5 which is 3 pH units removed from plasma and means approximately a thousandfold gradient for hydrogen ions.

The Link Between Lung and Kidney

It now remains to link together the role of the kidney and the lung in the overall management of varying hydrogen ion loads.

The lung is concerned with the excretion of the CO$_2$ produced as hydrogen ion is trapped by bicarbonate and converted into water. It is therefore concerned with keeping the equation shown here moving "from left to right".

The kidney is concerned with regenerating bicarbonate and so is concerned with keeping things moving "from right to left".

$$H^+ + HCO_3^- \rightarrow H_2CO_3 \rightarrow H_2O + CO_2$$

108

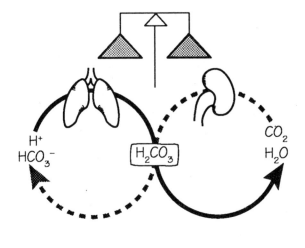

But the two organs are not pulling in opposite direction, rather they are yoked together in a continuum which may be drawn like a figure-of-eight.

In terms of laboratory study, this figure-of-eight is expressed by the Henderson Hasselbalch equation which links lung and kidney by expressing pH in terms of the lung (Pco_2) and the kidney (bicarbonate concentration).

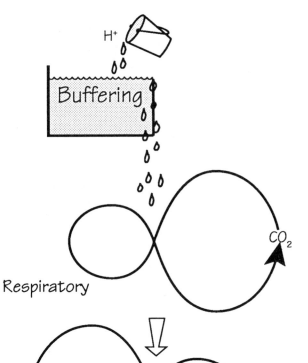

It works like this:

Buffering acts as a reservoir to "even out" the flow of hydrogen ions into the respiratory and renal mechanisms. It is virtually instantaneous.

The relatively rapid respiratory response emphasizes the shift of the carbonic acid buffer system towards the production of carbon dioxide (distorting the figure-eight).

The slower renal response then emphasizes bicarbonate recovery from the kidney (distorting the figure-eight in the opposite direction).

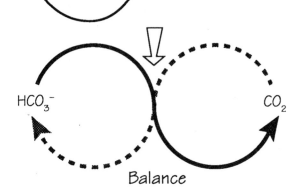

The end result is a re-establishment of the steady state with pH, Pco_2, and bicarbonate concentration all being in their normal range.

109

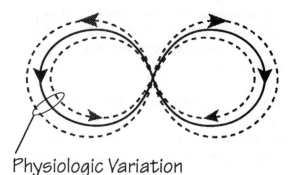

Physiologic Variation

In the normal events of physiological regulation, the distortion of this system in either direction is never great and pH variation is small.

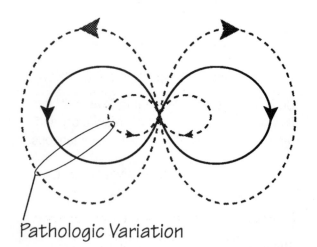

Pathologic Variation

Only in the catastrophes of abnormal events do the distortions become so large as to produce swings of pH that go well outside the acceptable limits and outside the ability of normal regulatory processes to correct them.

Failure of the lung or the kidney to fulfill their task in this regulatory system is often at the root of such distortions of pH regulation.

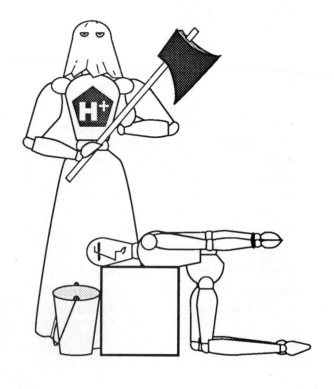

Clinical Examples of Disturbed H⁺ Handling

The major clinical threat is of overproduction of hydrogen ions. Acidosis is a more common problem than alkalosis.

Since the bicarbonate/carbonic acid buffer system is the most important indicator of the regulation of hydrogen ion concentration in the E.C.F., it is the most useful relationship to work with at a clinical level. It can be expressed in terms of the Henderson-Hasselbalch equation.

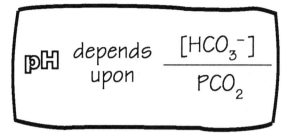

It will be recalled that for practical purposes, the equation can be rewritten in the fashion shown here to indicate that the carbonic acid level can be expressed in terms of P_{CO_2} and bicarbonate and that there is a fixed relationship between pH, bicarbonate concentration and P_{CO_2}.

This means that if any two of the three variables is measured then the third can be calculated.

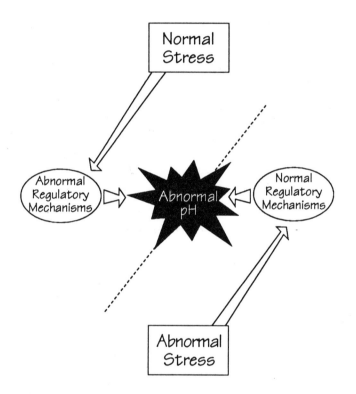

The normal pH "stresses" of everyday life are adequately handled by the physiologic mechanisms that have been described.

However,

1. The stress of an abnormal hydrogen ion load or

2. Disordered function of lungs or kidneys in the presence of a normal stress.

   Will lead to a breakdown of compensation.

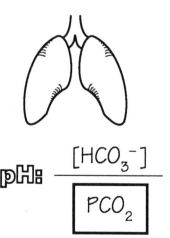

Respiratory Disturbances

In respiratory disturbances, therefore, the primary change is of the P_{CO_2}. This produces a change in pH and then a compensatory change in bicarbonate. To the extent that the respiratory problem is not reversed and to the extent that the renal compensation (bicarbonate loss or gain) is incomplete or delayed, so the pH will rise or fall.

The commonest presentation of a respiratory disturbance of pH is the acidosis of respiratory failure seen, for example, in a patient with an exacerbation of chronic bronchitis.

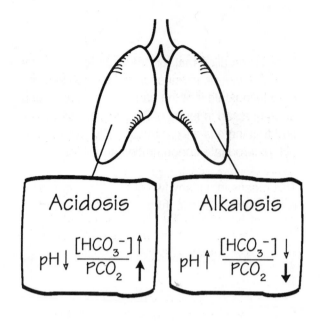

Acidosis

$$pH \downarrow \quad \frac{[HCO_3^-] \uparrow}{PCO_2} \uparrow$$

Alkalosis

$$pH \uparrow \quad \frac{[HCO_3^-] \downarrow}{PCO_2} \downarrow$$

Respiratory changes will produce changes in P_{CO_2} and compensatory changes of bicarbonate concentration will occur in the same direction, thus limiting the degree of the pH change. For example, in respiratory failure, the P_{CO_2} rises thus tending to lower the pH, but the bicarbonate concentration will also rise to compensate and thus correct the acidosis (at least in part).

In overventilation the P_{CO_2} falls and the reverse changes occur –respiratory alkalosis with compensating fall in bicarbonate.

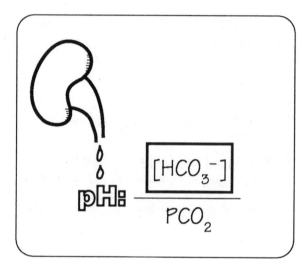

$$pH: \quad \frac{[HCO_3^-]}{PCO_2}$$

Metabolic Disturbances

Non-respiratory, or metabolic, events involve primary changes in the levels of bicarbonate with a compensatory respiratory response. Depending on the degree to which the stress continues and the compensation is incomplete, there will be changes of pH.

The limiting factor is the rate at which the kidney can manufacture or excrete bicarbonate.

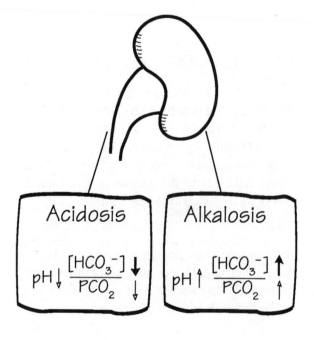

Acidosis

$$pH \downarrow \quad \frac{[HCO_3^-] \downarrow}{PCO_2} \downarrow$$

Alkalosis

$$pH \uparrow \quad \frac{[HCO_3^-] \uparrow}{PCO_2} \uparrow$$

The changes of pH, bicarbonate concentration and P_{CO_2} are shown here for metabolic problems.

It will be recognized that for a given shift of pH the bicarbonate concentration and P_{CO_2} change in the same direction, but for metabolic disturbances that direction is the opposite of what occurs in respiratory disturbances.

For a respiratory acidosis P_{CO_2} and bicarbonate concentration both rise, but for a metabolic acidosis they both fall.

	Respiratory	Metabolic
Acidosis pH↓	$\dfrac{[HCO_3^-]\,\uparrow}{PCO_2\,\uparrow}$	$\dfrac{[HCO_3^-]\,\downarrow}{PCO_2\,\downarrow}$
Alkalosis pH↓	$\dfrac{[HCO_3^-]\,\downarrow}{PCO_2\,\downarrow}$	$\dfrac{[HCO_3^-]\,\uparrow}{PCO_2\,\uparrow}$

In terms of the Henderson-Hasselbalch relationship it is clear that respiratory and metabolic effects look different.

The thick arrows in this table indicate the initial change, whilst the thin arrows indicate the physiologic response which attempts to correct the resulting pH change.

Thus, for example, a respiratory acidosis involves an initial rise of Pco_2 followed by a compensatory rise of bicarbonate which may be considered a compensatory metabolic alkalosis.

Similarly a metabolic alkalosis will be associated with a compensatory respiratory acidosis.

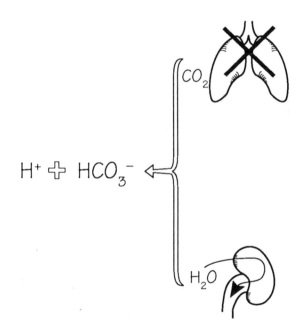

$$H^+ + HCO_3^-$$

Respiratory Acidosis

If the lungs are unable to excrete carbon dioxide, then of course, the E.C.F. is unable to handle hydrogen ions and a respiratory acidosis results, because the reaction cannot move from left to right as carbon dioxide accumulates.

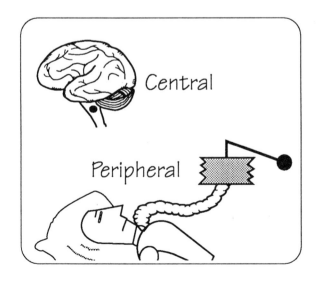

Respiratory Alkalosis

Alkalosis is generally a less common primary problem than acidosis.

Respiratory alkalosis occurs due to over-ventilation. Many causes can be listed but can be classified as central and peripheral. Central causes include the hyperventilation of anxiety or secondary to brain stem injury by disease or drugs. Peripheral causes include uncontrolled use of artificial ventilation.

Whatever the mechanism, the resultant fall of Pco_2 causes the pH to rise.

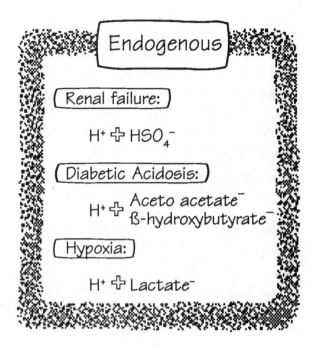

Endogenous

Renal failure:

$$H^+ + HSO_4^-$$

Diabetic Acidosis:

$$H^+ + \begin{array}{l} \text{Aceto acetate}^- \\ \text{ß-hydroxybutyrate}^- \end{array}$$

Hypoxia:

$$H^+ + \text{Lactate}^-$$

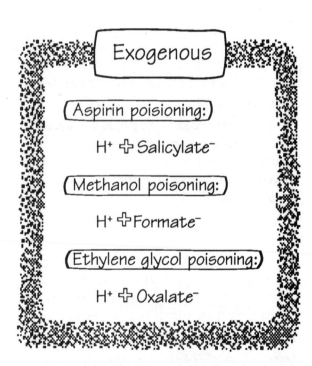

Exogenous

Aspirin poisioning:

$$H^+ + \text{Salicylate}^-$$

Methanol poisoning:

$$H^+ + \text{Formate}^-$$

Ethylene glycol poisoning:

$$H^+ + \text{Oxalate}^-$$

A Basic Rule

$$[\text{Anions}^-] \equiv [\text{Cations}^+]$$

Metabolic Acidosis

Metabolic acidosis may be due either to:
1) The retention of hydrogen ions produced by metabolic activity or
2) The loss of endogenously produced bicarbonate.

1. DUE TO RETENTION OF H⁺

Retention of H⁺ may occur in company with some anions not usually present in high concentration. Such situations may arise from "endogenous" disease processes or from loading by "exogenous" acids.

Accumulation of "endogenous" hydrogen ion will occur in association with a number of anions.

Thus in
1) Renal failure, anions such as phosphate and sulphate are retained.
2) Diabetic acidosis, anions such as acetoacetate and ß-hydroxybutyrate are retained.
3) Severe hypoxia, lactate is retained.

The presence of "exogenous" hydrogen ions is associated with accumulation of the accompanying anions which are not normal physiologic metabolites. Such anions include.

1) Salicylate, in acetyl salicylate (aspirin) overdose.
2) Formate, in methanol poisoning.
3) Oxalate, in ethylene glycol poisoning.

THE PLASMA ANION GAP

The accumulation of anions, either normal or abnormal will disturb the pattern of anions that are usually measured in the plasma. It is, of course, a physical and chemical reality that in the body fluids anions and cations must be present in equal concentrations. This applies to all body fluids including the plasma and the urine.

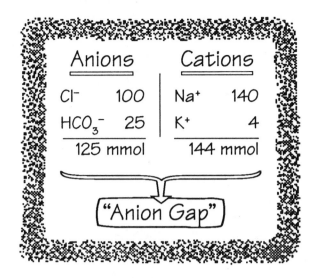

Normally the anions and cations in plasma are distributed as shown here, and you will recognize that they are apparently not present in equal concentration. This is, of course, because the missing anions are comprised of many different substances which we do not normally measure, but they are all present in small amounts and together make up the "anion gap".

They include sulphate, phosphate, anionic proteins and various organic anions.

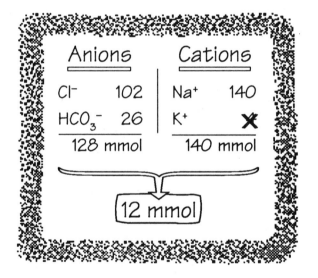

Because the potassium ion concentration is so small and will vary only a small amount it is, by convention, generally excluded when the anion gap is calculated.

Normally it is between 8 and 16 millimoles of unmeasured anions per litre.

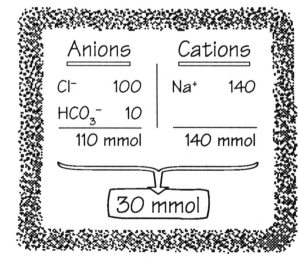

The unmeasured anions become significant, for example, in renal failure when hydrogen ions together with anions are retained. The retained anions are not measured, but greatly increase the anion gap.

Metabolic acidosis with an abnormally wide anion gap means an accumulation of anions which accompany the hydrogen ions. The anions may be those normally present, but in small amounts (e.g. phosphate, lactate) or those not normally present (e.g. salicylate).

As the hydrogen ions accumulate and cause the bicarbonate concentration to fall, the accompanying anions "fill the gap" that bicarbonate filled before.

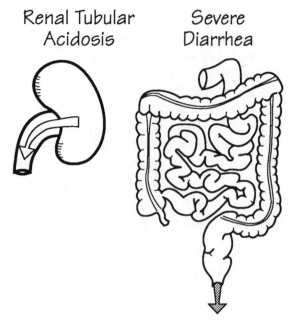

Renal Tubular
Acidosis

Severe
Diarrhea

2. METABOLIC ACIDOSIS DUE TO LOSS OF HCO$_3^-$

The depletion or removal of bicarbonate will cause the pH to fall just as surely as if free hydrogen ions were added.

Metabolic acidosis may be due to bicarbonate loss. This may be from the intestine, where losses from below the pylorus (severe small intestinal diarrhea) contain bicarbonate. Or it may be renal in origin where a failure of the tubules to generate or transport H$^+$ results in a failure to generate new bicarbonate and in some cases a failure to trap filtered bicarbonate. This is called renal tubular acidosis (RTA).

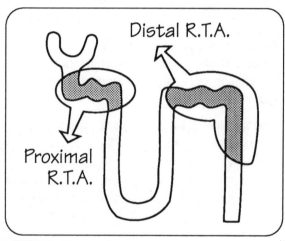

Distal R.T.A.

Proximal R.T.A.

Distal RTA results from a failure of the distal H$^+$ transport system probably due to a defect of H$^+$-ATP-ase. The urine cannot be acidified and urinary buffers cannot be saturated.

Proximal RTA results from a defect of proximal H$^+$ production or transport. There may be a defect of carbonic anhydrase or a problem with the Na$^+$/H$^+$ antiporter.

Failure to transport hydrogen ion or to generate it of course means a failure at a renal level to generate new bicarbonate.

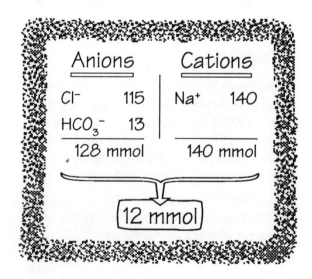

Anions		Cations	
Cl$^-$	115	Na$^+$	140
HCO$_3^-$	13		
128 mmol		140 mmol	

12 mmol

In these situations therefore pH can be viewed as falling because of the loss of bicarbonate anions. Since there is no accumulation of unmeasured anions, the anion gap has to be filled by something other than bicarbonate. The most readily available anion is, of course, chloride and the concentration of this anion increases to fill the gap left by the loss of bicarbonate.

This can be recognized by the presence of an acidosis with a normal plasma anion gap and hyperchloremia, and is often called "hyperchloremic acidosis".

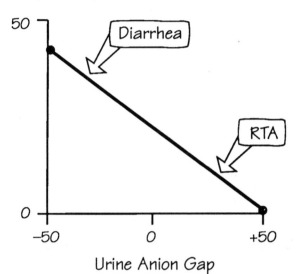

Urinary NH$_4^+$
(mmol/L)

Urine Anion Gap
(mmol/L)

THE URINARY ANION GAP

In patients with acidosis and a normal plasma anion gap, it may be clinically useful to measure the urinary anion gap which is expressed as urinary $([Na^+]+[K^+]) - [Cl^-]$.

The major anion in the urine is Cl^-.

The major cations in the urine are Na^+, K^+ and NH_4^+. Of these NH_4^+ is not usually measured.

The difference between measured cations and measured anions is therefore an index of the amount of NH_4^+ in the urine.

In metabolic acidosis, and with normal kidneys, NH_4^+ excretion will increase and the urine anion gap will become increasingly negative. This applies to small intestinal bicarbonate losses.

In metabolic acidosis due to renal failure or the common form of renal tubular acidosis (RTA) the urinary anion gap becomes increasingly positive.

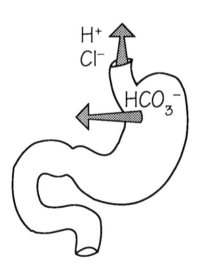

Metabolic Alkalosis

Metabolic alkalosis may be due to ingestion of absorbable alkali (such as sodium bicarbonate) or to loss of hydrogen ion due to vomiting. Since vomiting results in loss of chloride as well as hydrogen ion the striking rise of bicarbonate will go along with a severe depression of chloride.

Whether caused by direct loss of hydrogen ions or a rising bicarbonate, the final result is a rising pH.

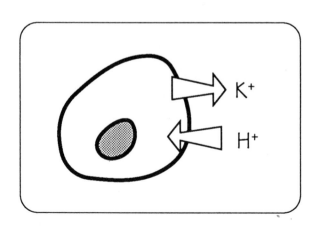

Vomiting also causes a loss of E.C.F. volume and of potassium. The former leads to aldosterone secretion which will add to the potassium loss at renal level. Hypokalemia exaggerates the alkalosis because as potassium leaves the cells to replace E.C.F. losses, it exchanges with hydrogen ion in the E.C.F. Thus a metabolic alkalosis is exaggerated by additional hypokalemic metabolic alkalosis due to movement of hydrogen ion into the I.C.F.

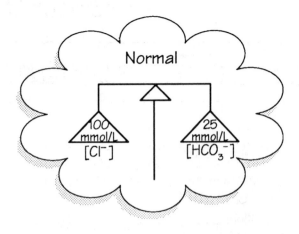

The Importance of Chloride

It has already been noted that hyperchloremic acidosis is seen when bicarbonate falls without the retention of any unmeasured anions.

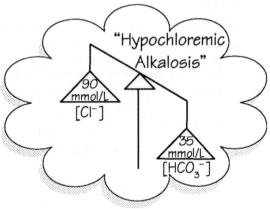

It is often not recognized that the converse is true. If the chloride concentration rises, then the bicarbonate concentration must fall (provided unmeasured anions remain constant). This will result in acidosis as an inevitable consequence of the fall in bicarbonate concentration. It can be seen clinically when inappropriately large amounts of isotonic sodium chloride are given intravenously. This is sometimes called "dilutional acidosis"

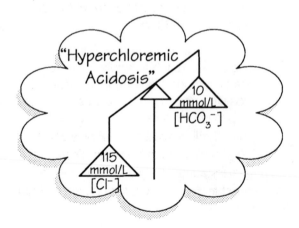

It will be apparent that chloride and bicarbonate will vary inversely with one another so long as the unmeasured anions do not change.

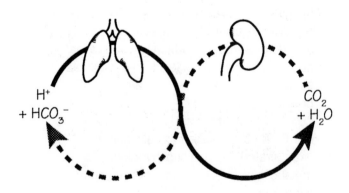

A Final Word

All disturbances of pH regulation include respiratory and metabolic components; one will initiate changes whilst the other will show a compensatory change. This is the essential concept linking the functions of lung and kidney and expressed by the Henderson Hasselbalch equation.

On the basis of this conceptual framework you should find the more detailed treatment of pH regulation in the literature easier to understand.

118

Chapter 9

The Regulation of Potassium

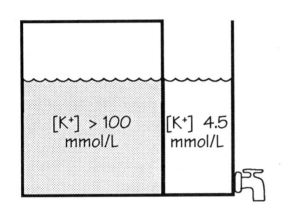

Most of the potassium in the body is within the I.C.F. Only a fraction is in the E.C.F., uniformly distributed through plasma and interstitial compartments.

The reference range for plasma potassium concentration is 3.5 to 5.0 mmol/L. Serum potassium concentration is slightly higher at 3.5 to 5.5 mmol/L.

Because the plasma potassium concentration is low, it will not vary appreciably with changes of total body water (unlike the situation with the predominantly extracellular sodium ion).

Changes of plasma potassium concentration reflect

1) Changes of total body potassium

2) Shifts of potassium into or out of the large intracellular pool.

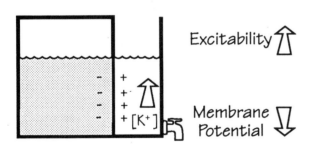

Although the concentration of potassium in the E.C.F. is small it is a critical determinant of the resting membrane potential of cells, which results largely from the leak of potassium from their interior.

If the concentration of potassium outside the cells rises, the membrane potential falls resulting in the membrane being more readily depolarised. This means a lower threshold for excitation of tissues such as nerve and muscle when the E.C.F. concentration of potassium rises.

Conversely it means a higher threshold for excitation when the E.C.F. concentration of potassium falls.

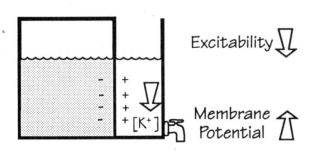

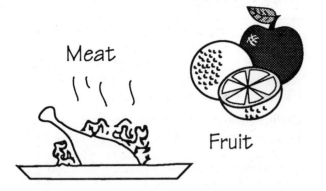

Dietary Potassium

Meat

Fruit

Intake

Potassium enters the body in the diet and is present in virtually all protein-containing foods, particularly meat.

On a North American diet the potassium intake is directly related to protein intake and is about 60 to 80 millimoles per day.

Although fruits and fruit juices are well known to be rich in potassium, they do not comprise the major source of this ion in a normal diet.

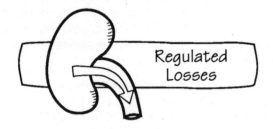

Regulated Losses

Output

Potassium leaves the body primarily via the kidney, which is the most important route because it is most open to physiologic regulation.

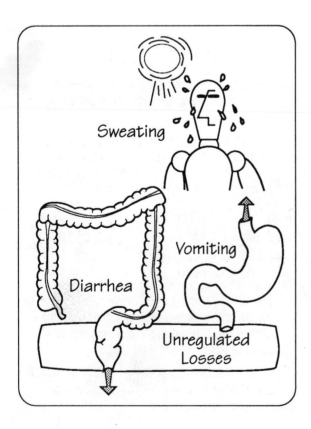

Sweating

Vomiting

Diarrhea

Unregulated Losses

However, potassium can leave the body in colonic fluid and via the sweat glands, routes which may be significant at times since the humoral regulator of potassium excretion (aldosterone) acts at these sites as well as on the renal tubule.

In normal situations, however, colon and skin are not of great importance in potassium regulation.

In abnormal states, losses from the intestine via diarrhea and vomiting may be very important. In this context all intestinal fluids are rich in potassium and their uncontrolled loss may be very large.

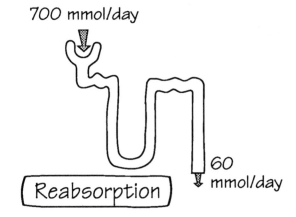

700 mmol/day

60 mmol/day

Reabsorption

Potassium and the Kidney

Because the plasma concentration of potassium is low, as compared with sodium, the amount filtered at the glomerulus is also low, about 700 millimoles per day, far less than the 25,000 millimoles of sodium that is filtered.

Normal subjects on a normal Canadian diet take in and excrete about 60 millimoles of potassium per day. Thus, with 700 millimoles filtered and only 60 millimoles excreted there must usually be net tubular reabsorption.

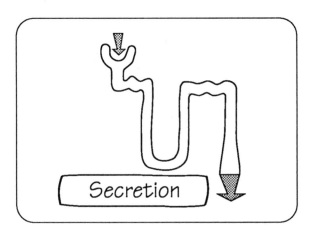

Secretion

Whilst this is the normal pattern, conditions can occur in which potassium excretion is higher than the filtered load of potassium. This must, of course, be an indication that the tubule is capable of potassium secretion as well as reabsorption.

Micropuncture studies have shown that most of the filtered potassium is reabsorbed in the proximal tubule (about 70%) and the thick ascending limb of the loop of Henle (about 20%).

The Proximal Tubule

The mechanisms operating in the proximal tubule are not fully understood but probably include these three.

1) In the early proximal tubule the lumen is slightly electronegative. Uphill (active) transport may be provided by a potassium pump in the luminal membrane.

2) In the late proximal tubule the lumen is slightly electropositive and this favours the movement of potassium across the wall via paracellular pathways.

3) The combination of "leaky" tight junctions and a very large transtubular flux of sodium and water is likely to carry potassium ions along with the outward flux of water and solutes from the proximal tubule.

Proximal reabsorption appears to be relatively fixed and does not vary to any degree with changing physiologic events.

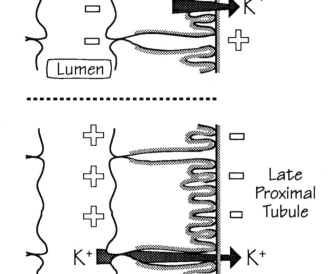

Early Proximal Tubule

K^+

Lumen

Late Proximal Tubule

K^+

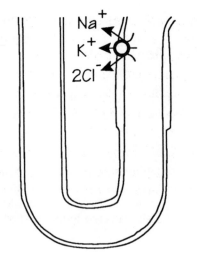

In the thick ascending limb of the loop of Henle, potassium leaves the tubule by a transcellular route. It crosses the luminal membrane using the $Na^+/K^+/2Cl^-$ cotransporter and can then cross the basolateral membrane down its concentration gradient. (see page 69)

As a result of these processes virtually all of the filtered potassium is reabsorbed by the end of the loop of Henle.

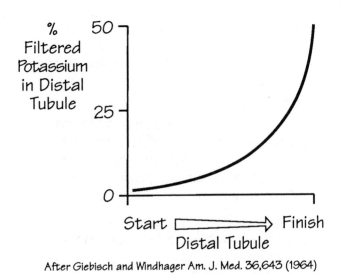

After Giebisch and Windhager Am. J. Med. 36,643 (1964)

The Distal Tubule

However, in the distal tubule potassium reappears to the extent that virtually all of the potassium appearing in the final urine in a normal subject is secreted into the distal tubule.

The initial assumption, therefore, was that after almost complete active reabsorption of potassium proximally there must be some secretory process in the distal tubule responsible for the reappearance of potassium at that site.

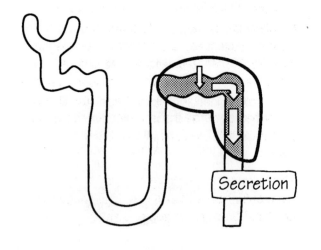

Since this secretion occurred at a part of the tubule where active sodium reabsorption was known to occur under the influence of aldosterone, it was considered that potassium was moving actively from cell to lumen by means of a pump mechanism that might be linked to sodium reabsorption. However the amount of sodium reabsorbed was much higher than the amount of potassium secreted.

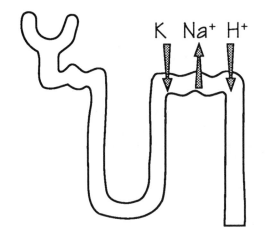

At this site much of the sodium is reabsorbed in exchange for actively secreted hydrogen ions and it was thought that potassium and hydrogen ions were competing in some way for the same transport system which in turn was linked to sodium transport in the reverse direction.

It is now recognized that no active luminal secretory process for potassium is present. The movement of potassium into the tubular lumen works like this:

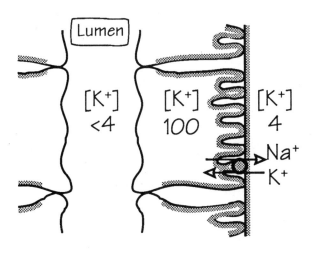

1) The Principal Cells

Within the principal cells of the distal system lies the mechanism responsible for the secretion of potassium into the urine.

The energy of this process is derived from the Na^+/K^+ ATP-ase in the basolateral membrane which powers the pump that maintains a high intracellular concentration of potassium and a low intracellular concentration of sodium.

This maintains a chemical gradient for potassium which favours its diffusion into the lumen.

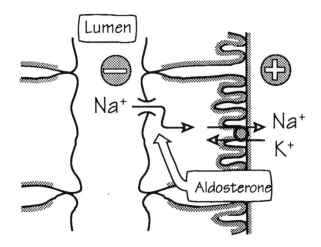

A second effect of the Na^+/K^+ pump at the basolateral membrane is to pump sodium out of the cell, maintaining a gradient favourable for the diffusion of sodium across the luminal membrane to enter the active transport system and move out into the interstitial space. This is enhanced by aldosterone which increases the permeability of the luminal membrane to sodium.

This movement of sodium from lumen to peritubular space results in a lumen negative electrical gradient (of about -50 mV).

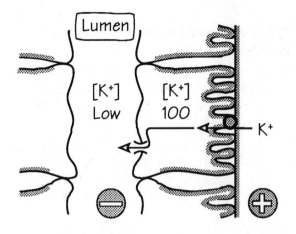

The electrical gradient, the concentration gradient for potassium and the fact that the luminal membrane is very permeable to potassium all result in the movement of potassium into the tubular lumen. In effect potassium is pumped into the base of the cell and then moves down the electrical and chemical gradients into the tubule.

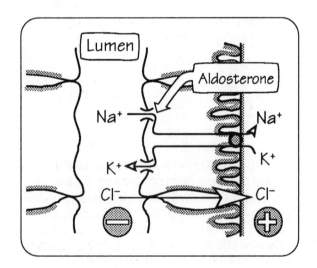

This process is moderated by aldosterone which increases the number of open sodium and potassium channels in the luminal membrane and thus increases the activity of the Na^+/K^+ pump at the basolateral membrane.

Aldosterone release from the adrenal gland is directly stimulated by increasing serum concentration of potassium and potassium secretion can be directly related to potassium intake.

The luminal negativity also leads to chloride reabsorption through the paracellular pathway.

2) The Intercalated Cells

In the cortical collecting duct most cells are Principal cells, but in the medullary collecting duct the number of Intercalated cells predominates.

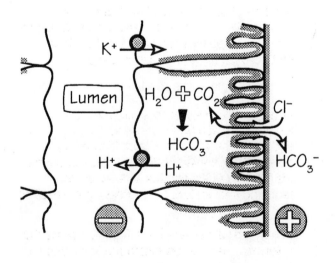

These have a major role in the pumping out of hydrogen ions against a concentration gradient, acidifying the urine and maximizing the ability of the nephron to dispose of hydrogen ions and make fresh bicarbonate.

These cells also provide a distal reabsorptive pathway for potassium via the activity of an active potassium transport system in the luminal membrane.

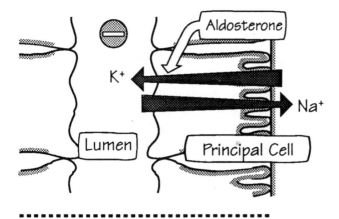

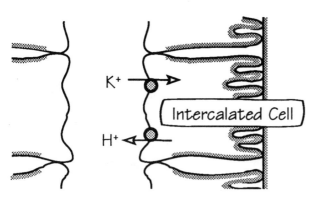

Tubular management of potassium can be summarised as follows:

1) Proximal potassium reabsorption is very nearly complete by the end of the loop of Henle, and a fixed property of the tubule, not open to independent regulation.

2) The distal system represents the only part of the nephron that can provide regulated management of potassium and respond to the need of the body as a whole to lose or gain potassium.

There are two intrinsic concerns with this regulatory process.

i) Potassium secretion by the Principal cells depends upon the potential gradients produced by active sodium reabsorption and is thus "subservient" to it.

ii) Hydrogen ions pumped out by the intercalated cells will diminish this potential gradient and thus limit the capacity to excrete a potassium load.

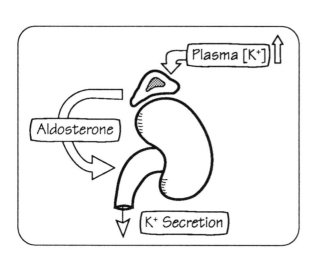

It is therefore clear that in many situations potassium secretion is determined by the priorities of sodium reabsorption and hydrogen ion secretion, however the rate of potassium secretion in the distal tubule can be directly influenced by the plasma potassium because an increased plasma concentration of potassium can directly stimulate aldosterone release from the adrenal gland. This is a direct reaction which is independent of the renin-angiotensin-aldosterone system.

In states of sodium depletion aldosterone release will, of course, be renin-dependent and is the major pathway by which distal tubular reabsorption of sodium is increased.

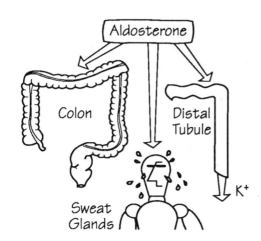

Whatever the stimulus to its secretion, aldosterone results in increasing tubular sodium reabsorption and thus increasing potassium secretion. Aldosterone also acts on the large intestine and the sweat glands, reducing sodium loss but increasing potassium loss by these routes.

In patients with severe renal failure, loss via the colon may be an important factor in limiting the degree of hyperkalemia.

125

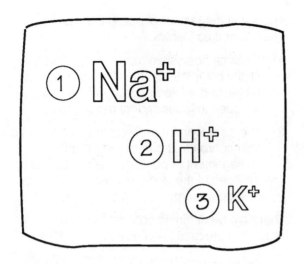

It is clear that the kidney handles sodium, hydrogen, and potassium ions in a closely linked manner. As a general rule, for the whole organism, renal handling of sodium seems to take priority over regulation of the other cations. Regulation of sodium balance will often occur at the expense of hydrogen or potassium ions when external stresses demand it.

Similarly, provided sodium balance is satisfied, pH regulation often will be at the expense of E.C.F. potassium regulation.

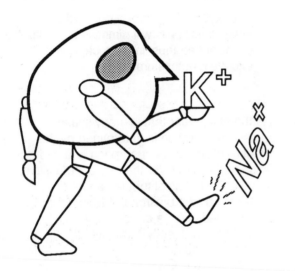

Presumably the reason for potassium regulation tending to be lower on the list of priorities as far as the E.C.F. is concerned is that potassium is predominantly the property of the I.C.F.

It is the cells that have an efficient pump to keep potassium inside and sodium outside and therefore it is the cells as a whole that contain and regulate the bulk of body potassium.

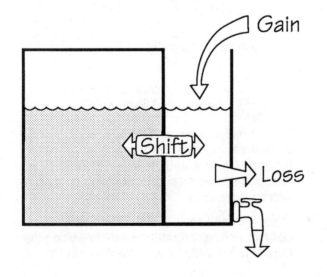

Clinical Examples of Disturbed Potassium Metabolism

Changes in the plasma potassium concentration may reflect

1) Loss or gain of total body potassium

2) Shifts of potassium into or out of the cells, often dependent upon reciprocal movements of hydrogen ions.

3) A combination of the two.

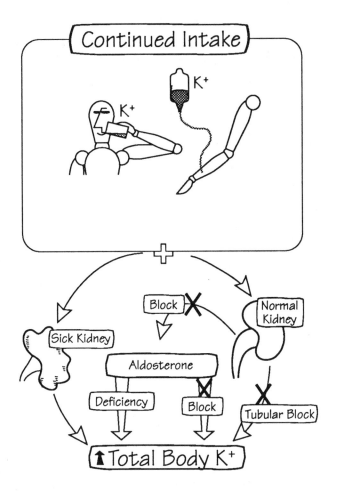

Hyperkalemia

Hyperkalemia is a potentially life-threatening metabolic emergency. It has two basic mechanisms.

1) INCREASED BODY POTASSIUM

In the presence of a continued intake of potassium the following factors may cause potassium retention.

a) Intrinsic renal disease with impaired capacity to secrete potassium.

b) Deficiency of aldosterone due to adrenal dysfunction.

c) Deficiency of the stimulus of angiotensin II to aldosterone production caused by angiotensin converting enzyme inhibitors (e.g. captopril).

d) Inhibition of the effect of aldosterone upon the distal tubule e.g. by the competitive inhibitor spironolactone.

e) Direct inhibition of sodium transport in the distal tubule by drugs such as amiloride and triamterene.

2) A SHIFT FROM CELLS TO E.C.F.

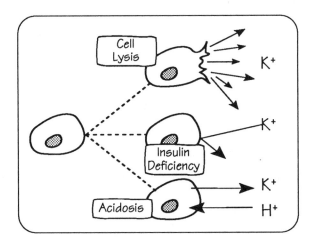

This will cause hyperkalemia without any increase in total body potassium. Important causes are

a) Severe systemic acidosis. Potassium leaves the cells in exchange for hydrogen ions which bind to intracellular buffers.

b) The insulin deficiency of diabetes mellitus, which prevents the normal effect of insulin in favouring the uptake of potassium by cells.

c) Massive release of potassium from damaged cells e.g. Rhabdomyolysis.

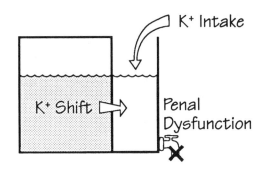

In practice there may often be more than one factor leading to an elevated plasma concentration of potassium.

Patients with renal dysfunction are always at greater risk than those with normal kidneys.

127

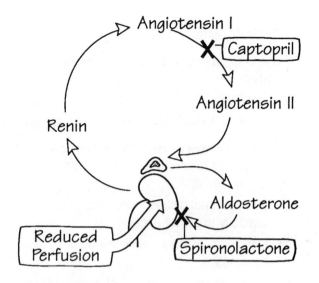

An example of such a clinical "mixture" is the inadvertent coincidental use of captopril and spironolactone in a diabetic with persistent heart failure and mild renal failure due to reduced "effective forward flow".

Such patients may also have a sluggish aldosterone response to hyperkalemia ("idiopathic hypoaldosteronism").

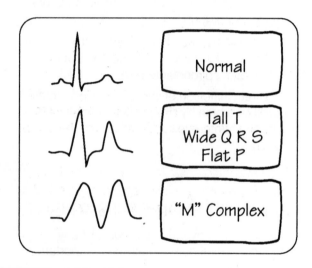

Clinically, hyperkalemia produces:

Weakness and irritable "twitchy" muscles
Fearfulness and parasthesiae
Cardiac arrhythmias progressing to ventricular fibrillation.

The EKG may show a sequence of changes as the plasma concentration of potassium rises; they can result in effective cardiac standstill at plasma concentration of potassium above 7.5-8.0 millimoles per litre.

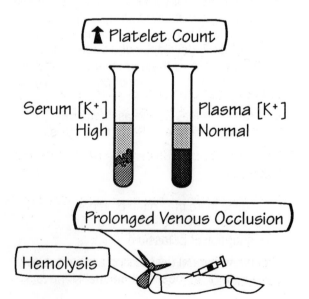

A "false" elevation of concentration of potassium in the serum may occur if the platelet count is very high since potassium is extruded from platelets trapped in a blood clot. In such situations the plasma potassium will be normal.

Similarly the prolonged occlusion of veins with a tourniquet can cause a false elevation of the plasma concentration of potassium due to purely local factors.

Hemolysis of blood after venepuncture, or delayed separation of cells and plasma may also give false plasma levels.

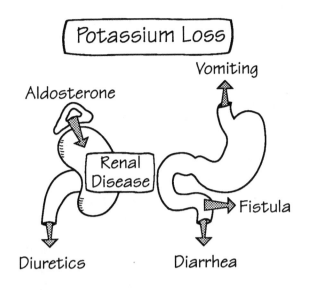

Potassium Loss

Vomiting

Aldosterone

Renal Disease

Fistula

Diuretics   Diarrhea

Hypokalemia

1) DUE TO A LOSS OF TOTAL BODY POTASSIUM

a) From the intestine due to vomiting, diarrhea or a surgical fistula.

b) From the kidney due to renal disease, diuretic administration or increased aldosterone production.

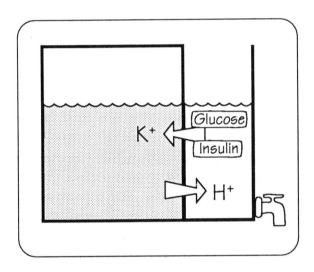

K^+

Glucose

Insulin

H^+

2) DUE TO A SHIFT FROM E.C.F. TO CELLS

Hypokalemia may be the result of a shift of potassium into the I.C.F. This is usually due to a primary alkalotic state or due to the correction of high blood sugar in diabetics with the use of insulin.

In alkalosis hydrogen ions leave the cells as part of the mechanism for correcting the E.C.F. pH and in doing so exchange for potassium.

Clinically, hypokalemia produces:

Severe weakness
Tetany
Cardiac arrhythmias

EKG changes are not as dramatic as in hyperkalemia and include ST depression, flat T waves and marked U waves.

The effects of digitalis become more marked in hypokalemia.

"Periodic paralysis" can be due to sudden shifts of potassium into the cells. Its mechanism is not understood and it is very rare.

Prolonged hypokalemia can cause secondary renal tubular damage which may be permanent.

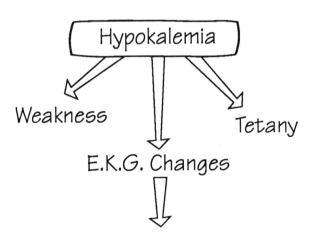

Hypokalemia

Weakness

Tetany

E.K.G. Changes

Increased digitalis effect

Chapter 10

The Regulation of Calcium and Phosphate

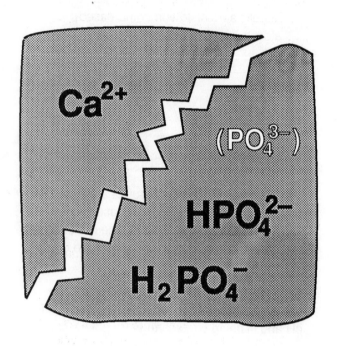

There is more calcium than any other cation in the human body, amounting to about 25,000 millimoles (1 kilogram) for an average man. Almost all of it is within the structure of bone, in company with phosphate.

Both calcium and phosphorus also have important intracellular roles, with phosphorus having particular importance because of its function in storing energy in organic phosphate compounds such as adenosine triphosphate (ATP).

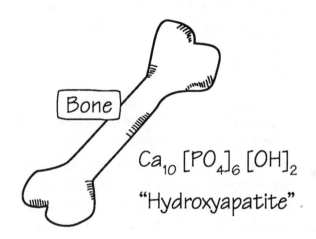

In their inorganic forms calcium and phosphate are locked together in the crystalline structure of bone. For this reason, it is impossible to consider calcium as an extracellular cation without considering phosphate anions at the same time.

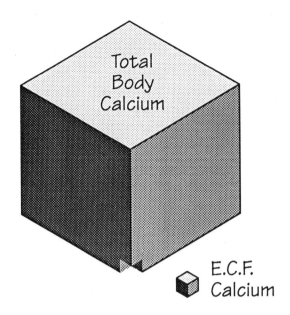

Total Body Calcium

E.C.F. Calcium

Precise regulation of calcium concentration in the E.C.F. is demanded because of the effects of extracellular calcium on nerve and muscle function (both skeletal and myocardial).

This poses problems because less than 1% of the total body calcium is in the E.C.F., the rest being within the bone. In spite of this wide difference in distribution, the E.C.F. calcium concentration remains precisely regulated.

Normal Plasma Calcium:	2.1 - 2.6 mmol/L (8.5 - 10.5 mg/dL)
50% is: Ca^{2+}	50% is: CaPr
1.25 mmol/L (5 mg/dL)	1.25 mmol/L (5 mg/dL)

E.C.F. Calcium

Within the E.C.F., calcium exists in two forms:

1) Free, ionized calcium

2) Bound calcium, predominantly attached to proteins, particularly albumin. A small amount is bound in a complex form with organic acids.

In the plasma compartment only half the calcium exists as free ionized calcium. The other half is bound to albumin, or complexed.

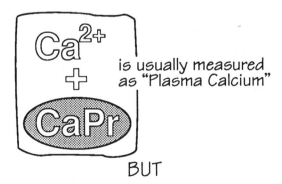

Ca^{2+} + CaPr is usually measured as "Plasma Calcium"

BUT

Only Ca^{2+} is physiologically important

It is the ionized calcium that is physiologically important, although in most clinical settings it is total plasma calcium that is measured.

The reference range for total calcium is 2.1 to 2.6 millimoles per litre (8.5 to 10.5 mg/dl).

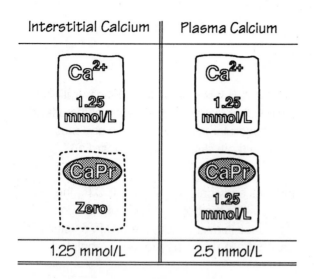

Interstitial Calcium	Plasma Calcium
Ca^{2+} 1.25 mmol/L	Ca^{2+} 1.25 mmol/L
CaPr Zero	CaPr 1.25 mmol/L
1.25 mmol/L	2.5 mmol/L

In the interstitial fluid compartment, where albumin concentrations are small, the calcium is predominantly in the ionized form, in equilibrium with the calcium ion concentration in the plasma.

Thus the total plasma calcium is approximately twice the concentration of interstitial calcium.

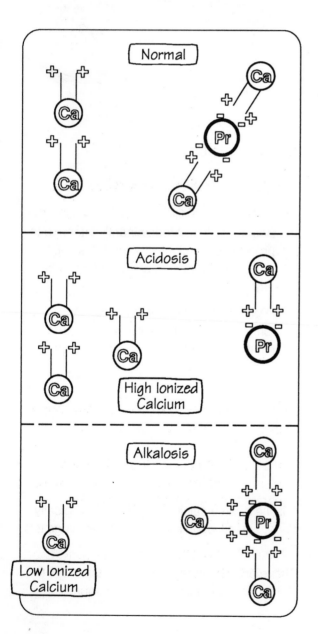

The Effect of pH Changes

It is important to remember that the degree of protein binding of calcium in the plasma will vary. In particular the binding is dependent upon pH, since the number of negative charges on protein molecules varies with changes of hydrogen ion concentration.

Thus the more acidic the plasma becomes, the fewer negatively charged binding sites will be available to fix calcium. So the free calcium ions will tend to rise.

Conversely the less acidic the plasma the more calcium ions will be protein bound. In states of alkalosis the amount of free calcium will fall.

This is important to clinicians who may see signs of hypocalcemia occurring in alkalotic patients whose total plasma calcium is normal, but whose free ionized calcium has fallen.

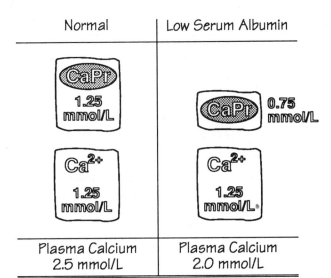

Normal	Low Serum Albumin
CaPr 1.25 mmol/L	CaPr 0.75 mmol/L
Ca²⁺ 1.25 mmol/L	Ca²⁺ 1.25 mmol/L
Plasma Calcium 2.5 mmol/L	Plasma Calcium 2.0 mmol/L

In patients with a low serum albumin the total plasma calcium will be low but the free ionized calcium will be normal.

Such patients will have no signs or symptoms of hypocalcemia, because these depend upon the ionized calcium concentration and not the total calcium concentration.

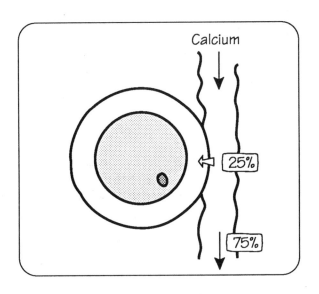

Calcium Absorption

Calcium enters the body via the intestine.

About 25 millimoles is ingested each day, but only about 25% of this is absorbed, the rest appearing in the feces.

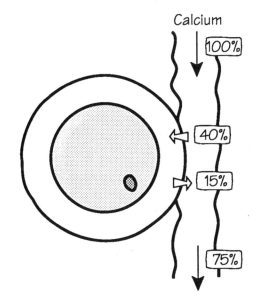

A 25% figure for absorption in the intestine is not quite accurate.

In fact about 40% of the intake is absorbed, but an amount, equal to about 15% of the intake, is secreted into the intestine as part of the digestive juices.

This results in a balance that is equivalent to only 25% absorption.

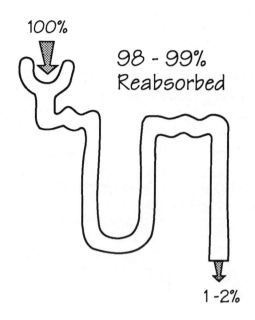

100%

98 - 99% Reabsorbed

1 -2%

Some calcium can leave the E.C.F. via the kidney. Ionized calcium is freely filtered by the renal glomerulus (while protein-bound calcium is not).

Most of what is filtered is reabsorbed by the tubule, only about 1-2% of the filtered calcium being lost in the final urine.

Total urinary losses are about 4-6 millimoles per day, which is equal to the daily net intestinal absorption.

Thus normal adults are in balance, with an intake of about 25 millimoles per day and a combined fecal and urinary loss of about 25 millimoles per day.

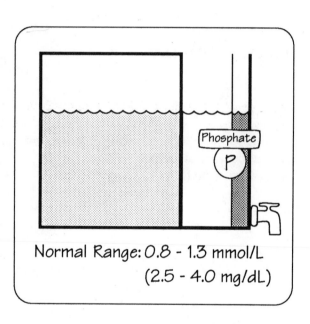

Phosphate
P

Normal Range: 0.8 - 1.3 mmol/L
(2.5 - 4.0 mg/dL)

E.C.F. Phosphate

Inorganic phosphate exists in the E.C.F. in two major forms, but the amount of phosphate present is usually expressed in terms of elemental phosphorus (P).

In the cells, of course, phosphorus also exists in organic forms such as ATP.

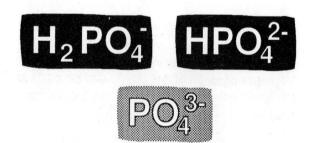

$H_2PO_4^-$ HPO_4^{2-}

PO_4^{3-}

The two major forms of phosphate are monohydrogen phosphate (HPO_4^{2-}) and dihydrogen phosphate ($H_2PO_4^-$).

Although a third form of phosphate (PO_4^{3-}) occurs, at physiologic levels of pH this form does not exist.

In the clinical setting the term "phosphate" is often used to refer to any of these forms indiscriminately.

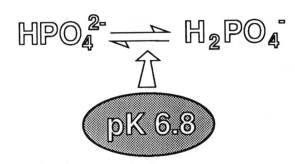

The relationship between the two major anionic forms of phosphate is determined by the pH of the E.C.F. The pH at which the two forms are in equilibrium is 6.8; that is, the reaction has a pK of 6.8.

Thus at a pH of 6.8 the concentration of monohydrogen phosphate equals the concentration of dihydrogen phosphate.

This means that at pH 6.8

$$[HPO_4^{2-}] \equiv [H_2PO_4^-]$$

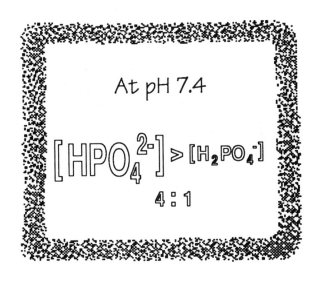

At the pH of extracellular fluid (7.4) about 80% of phosphate will exist as monohydrogen phosphate and 20% as dihydrogen phosphate.

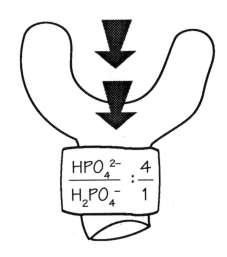

Urinary Phosphate

Phosphate is filtered at the glomerulus and in the filtrate the ratio of monohydrogen phosphate to dihydrogen phosphate is the same as in the plasma.

135

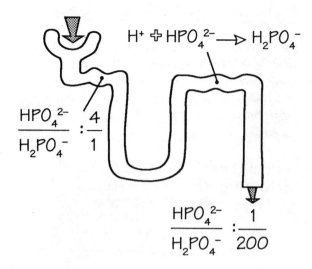

$$H^+ + HPO_4^{2-} \longrightarrow H_2PO_4^-$$

$$\frac{HPO_4^{2-}}{H_2PO_4^-} : \frac{4}{1}$$

$$\frac{HPO_4^{2-}}{H_2PO_4^-} : \frac{1}{200}$$

But as the filtrate moves down into the distal tubule the filtered phosphate acts as a buffer which traps hydrogen ions as they are pumped out of the tubular cells into the lumen.

As this continues the ratio between mono- and dihydrogen phosphate changes.

In very acid urine (pH about 4.5) with almost all phosphate buffering power saturated, dihydrogen phosphate may be up to two hundred times the concentration of monohydrogen phosphate.

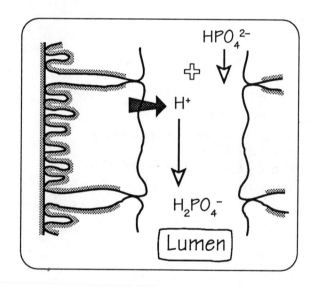

The relatively large amount of filtered phosphate allows a surplus of phosphate to be available for excretion through the renal tubule. On its way out in the urine this becomes the single most important buffer for "titratable acid" in the urine (see Chapter 8).

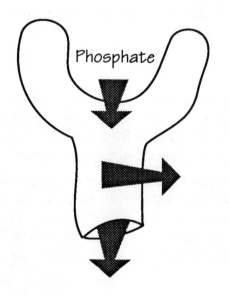

Reabsorption of filtered phosphate by the tubule occurs, but the reabsorptive capacity is normally at a low level so that changes in plasma phosphate levels (and thus in filtered phosphate) can change excretion markedly.

Changes in glomerular function can also alter plasma phosphate markedly.

In normal circumstances there is plenty of filtered phosphate escaping reabsorption in the tubule and available to buffer secreted hydrogen ions. Thus the kidney plays an important role in determining plasma phosphate levels.

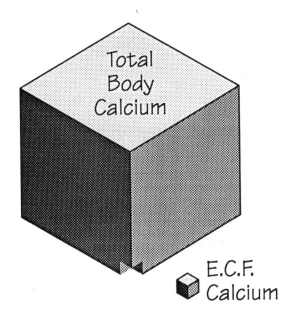

E.C.F. Calcium

Calcium and Phosphate

Because the E.C.F. concentration of calcium is small in relation to total body calcium, and because it has such marked physiological effects, it is important to understand the intricate mechanisms which have evolved to ensure that this narrow range is not violated.

A few millimoles lost or gained from the vast body store of calcium is neither here nor there, but a few millimoles lost or gained from the E.C.F. pool of calcium may be critical to survival, since ionized calcium is a vital determinant of membrane excitability.

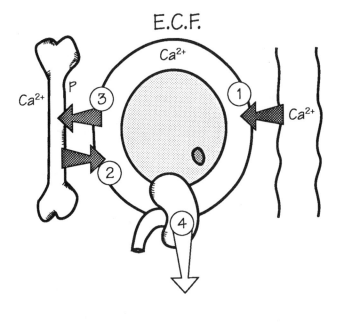

Clearly calcium can enter the E.C.F. in two ways:

1) By absorption from the intestine

2) By release from the store in bone

And it can leave the E.C.F.

3) By entering the bone

4) By excretion in the urine.

These facts underlie the mechanisms for regulation of E.C.F. calcium concentration.

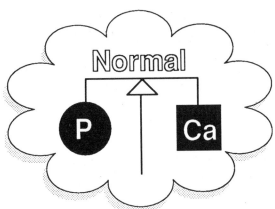

Clinically, the intimate relationship between calcium and phosphate has been expressed in terms of the product of the concentrations of the two in the plasma (the "solubility product").

Normally this product remains roughly constant. If it rises then calcium and phosphate will tend to precipitate out of solution, probably mainly into bone but sometimes (with abnormally high products) into soft tissues.

If One Goes Up...

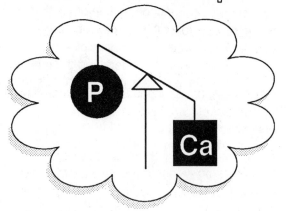

Ordinarily if the phosphate concentration rises the calcium concentration will fall, and vice versa. A reciprocal relationship therefore exists between calcium and phosphate on a direct physico-chemical basis. This relationship forms a background against which other regulatory processes will act.

...the Other Goes Down

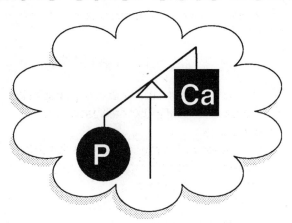

This reciprocal relationship is seen most obviously with elevations of E.C.F. phosphate concentration and it is important to note that many more complex factors come into play to determine the precise relationship between calcium and phosphate in any given situation.

Regulators

① Parathyroid Hormone

② Vitamin D

The two major factors which regulate calcium and phosphate concentrations are both humoral.

They are:

1) Parathyroid hormone

2) Vitamin D

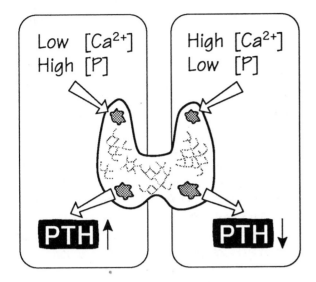

Parathyroid Hormone

Parathyroid hormone (PTH) is a peptide hormone secreted by the four parathyroid glands in the neck.

Secretion is increased by a fall of plasma ionized calcium concentration and decreased by a rise of plasma ionized calcium concentration.

Primary changes of plasma phosphate concentration will also modulate parathyroid hormone secretion presumably through their effects upon plasma calcium concentration.

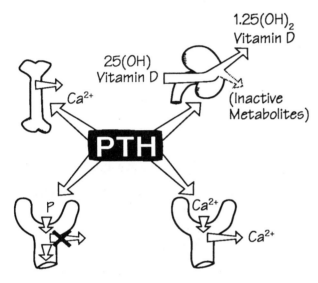

Parathyroid hormone probably has four main actions:

1) Release of calcium from bone (in the presence of Vitamin D).
2) Increase in renal tubular loss of phosphate.
3) Increase in renal tubular reabsorption of calcium.
4) Stimulation of the production of $1:25(OH)_2$ cholecalciferol rather than inactive metabolites of Vitamin D.

Vitamin D

Vitamin D is a steroid hormone (cholecalciferol) derived from precursors either ingested in the diet or produced by ultraviolet light acting upon the skin.

In the liver cholecalciferol is hydroxylated at the 25 position, a process not regulated by calcium or phosphate levels in the serum.

In the kidney further hydroxylation occurs and $1\text{-}\alpha$-hydroxylation produces "active Vitamin D" - $1:25(OH)_2$ cholecalciferol.

This step is stimulated by:

1) Low serum phosphate
2) Low serum calcium
3) PTH

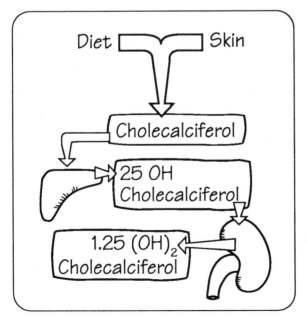

139

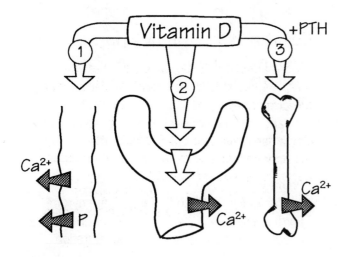

Activated Vitamin D probably has three main actions.

1) It enhances calcium and phosphate absorption from the intestine.
2) It enhances renal tubular calcium reabsorption.
3) It enhances calcium release from bone (in the presence of PTH).

Other actions may include renal phosphate retention, a direct role in bone mineralisation in certain situations (somewhat in conflict with 3 above) and possibly a direct suppressive effect upon PTH release. All these other actions remain incompletely worked out.

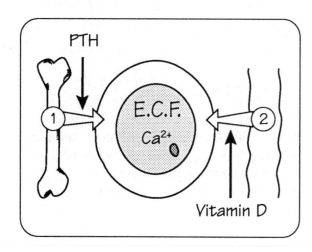

It is probably acceptable to simplify the actions of Vitamin D and PTH in the following way.

1) The major effect of PTH is to release calcium from the bone.
2) The major effect of Vitamin D is to enhance calcium transport across the intestinal wall.

Having said this, however, it is important to emphasize that these two hormones are complementary in their role as regulators of plasma calcium and phosphate levels.

The full effects of one do not occur without the coincident presence of the other.

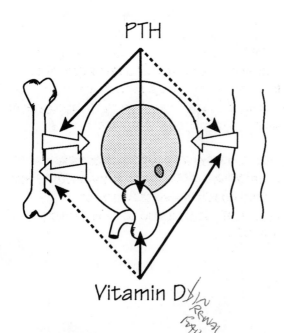

The precise nature and degree of collaboration between PTH and Vitamin D is still being unravelled but it is more complex than has been shown here and has been a fascinating story of modern biochemical research.

140

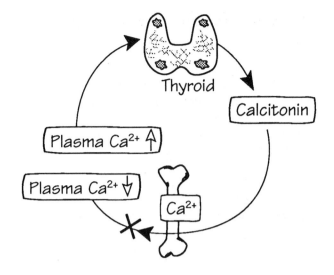

Calcitonin

A word about calcitonin, which is a peptide hormone secreted by the parafollicular cells of the thyroid gland.

Calcitonin lowers the E.C.F. calcium by reducing the release of calcium from bone. Its secretion is probably regulated directly by serum calcium concentrations. Its role in calcium regulation appears to be minor in man.

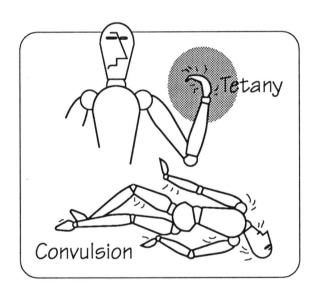

Some Clinical Issues

1) Hypocalcemia

A low plasma ionized calcium produces neuromuscular signs and symptoms. The best known sign is tetany characterized by muscle cramps involving the hands and feet. Sometimes convulsions may occur.

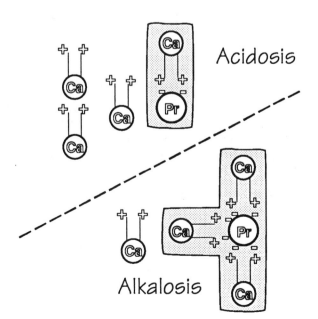

Tetany can occur without a measured fall in total serum calcium if a sudden rise in pH occurs, thus suddenly increasing the degree to which calcium is bound to proteins.

This may occur if metabolic acidosis is corrected too rapidly by the intravenous infusion of bicarbonate. It also occurs when hyperventilation leads to acute respiratory alkalosis.

141

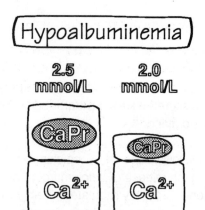

Hypoalbuminemia

2.5 mmol/L   2.0 mmol/L

CaPr   CaPr

Ca^{2+} Ca^{2+}

It is important to re-emphasize that a low total calcium concentration can occur with hypoalbuminemia without a low ionized calcium. In this situation therefore there are no signs or symptoms that would suggest hypocalcemia.

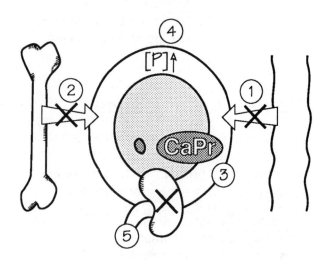

Amongst the causes of a low plasma ionized calcium concentration are:

1) Failure to absorb calcium from the intestine (e.g. Vitamin D deficiency, malabsorption).

2) Failure to release calcium from bone (e.g. PTH deficiency).

3) Increased calcium binding (e.g. alkalosis).

4) Hyperphosphatemia (e.g. renal failure).

5) Renal failure (failure to hydroxylate Vitamin D).

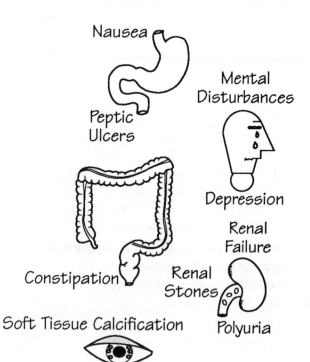

Nausea

Peptic Ulcers

Mental Disturbances

Depression

Constipation

Renal Stones

Renal Failure

Polyuria

Soft Tissue Calcification

2) Hypercalcemia

Hypercalcemia causes disordered intestinal motility, disturbances of higher cerebral function and renal damage (due to a direct toxic effect of calcium on the renal tubule).

Rapidly developing severe hypercalcemia produces profound polyuria, cerebral disturbances and disturbed cardiac function.

Prolonged hypercalcemia can lead to deposition of calcium salts in soft tissues. This may be seen as a ring at the edge of the cornea. Prolonged hypercalcemia can also lead to the formation of kidney stones.

142

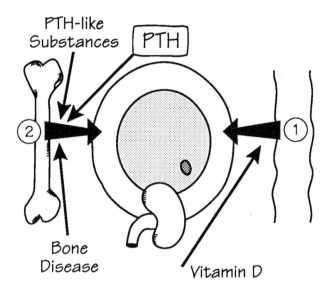

PTH-like Substances

PTH

Bone Disease

Vitamin D

Some causes of hypercalcemia are:

1) Increased intestinal absorption of calcium
    a) Due to an excess of Vitamin D
    b) Due to an increased sensitivity to normal amounts of Vitamin D (e.g. sarcoidosis).

2) Increased release of calcium from bone
    a) Due to the action of PTH (e.g. parathyroid tumors)
    b) Due to disease of the bone (e.g. metastatic cancer, multiple myeloma)
    c) Due to the action of PTH-like substances released from tumours (e.g. carcinoma of the bronchus).

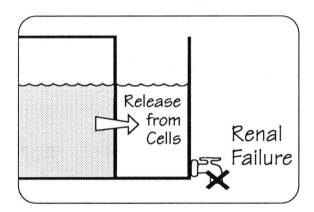

Release from Cells

Renal Failure

3) Hyperphosphatemia

A high phosphate level in the E.C.F. is usually due to renal failure which limits phosphate excretion. Occasionally it will occur in association with massive cell lysis (releasing phosphate from the cells), for example in hemolysis, and leukemia. It also occurs in diabetic coma.

The major effect of persistent hyperphosphatemia is the deposition of "calcium phosphate" in soft tissues. It will also produce "reciprocal" hypocalcemia.

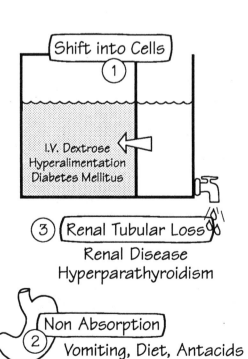

Shift into Cells

I.V. Dextrose
Hyperalimentation
Diabetes Mellitus

3) Renal Tubular Loss
Renal Disease
Hyperparathyroidism

Non Absorption
Vomiting, Diet, Antacids

4) Hypophosphatemia

Causes of hypophosphatemia include:

1) Shift of phosphate into cells along with dextrose during the rapid correction of diabetic ketoacidosis or in association with intravenous hyperalimentation.

2) Failure of intestinal absorption due to poor diet, alcoholism, vomiting or the use of phosphate-binding antacids.

3) Renal tubular loss in association with renal disease or secondary to hyperparathyroidism.

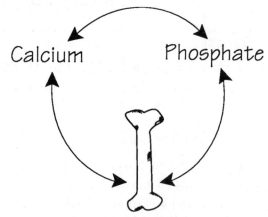

Calcium   Phosphate

5) Metabolic Bone Disease

It is evident that calcium and phosphate metabolism cannot be considered without recognising its close linkage to the behaviour of bone. For this reason long-standing disorders of regulation of calcium and phosphate may become clinically apparent as disease of bone.

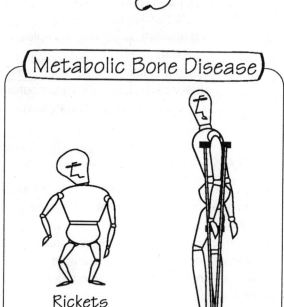

Metabolic Bone Disease

Rickets

Osteomalacia

The failure to mineralize bone results in striking disability because of an inadequate skeleton. This is most commonly due to a deficiency of Vitamin D, or a failure in its activation. Occasionally it may be due to calcium or phosphate deficiency.

In the growing child, a failure to mineralize bone results in the picture of rickets with characteristic deformities of growing bones. In the adult, it presents as osteomalacia with pathological "pseudofractures" of weight-bearing bones with pain and a characteristic "waddling" walk.

The underlying defect of calcium metabolism is reflected by a low plasma calcium which often leads to stimulation of the parathyroid glands and resultant "secondary" hyperparathyroidism.

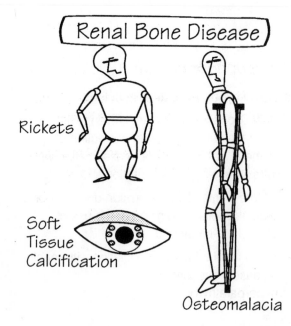

Renal Bone Disease

Rickets

Soft Tissue Calcification

Osteomalacia

The bone disease of long-standing renal failure is an example of the complexities of calcium and phosphate regulation. It presents as the clinical picture of rickets or osteomalacia often with associated soft tissue calcification. Factors which are involved include:

1) Failure to hydroxylate Vitamin D
2) Persistent hyperphosphatemia
3) Metabolic acidosis with consequent loss of calcium from bone in exchange for hydrogen ions
4) Secondary hyperparathyroidism
5) The replacement of calcium in bone by aluminum in patients being treated with aluminum hydroxide as a phosphate binder in prolonged renal failure treated by dialysis

144

Chapter 11

Some Therapeutic Guidelines

Treating disorders of fluids and electrolytes should be an exercise in applied physiology rather than the use of a "recipe book" approach. Some specific notes on therapy have been given in previous chapters, and here the discussion will be confined to some general principles which should encourage confidence that fluid therapy is not a great mystery but can be planned safely and logically using the basic concepts developed in this book. A few specific therapeutic problems will be discussed but no attempt will be made to provide a comprehensive guide and the reader is referred to more advanced texts for this purpose.

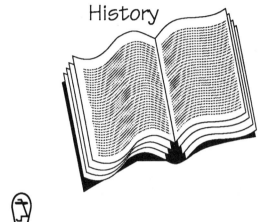

History

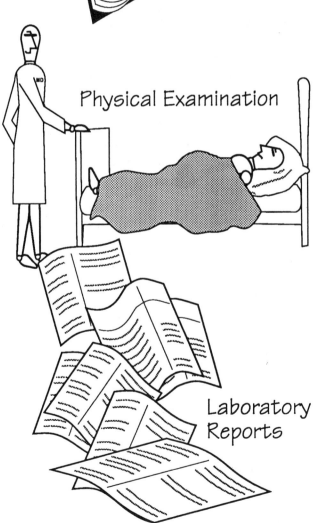

Physical Examination

Laboratory Reports

Getting Organized

In planning fluid and electrolyte management it is important to avoid the common temptation to start with laboratory data.

It is best to begin with a careful review of the history preceding the patient's current problems.

Physical examination should then be as careful as it would be in any other clinical situation.

Only when these steps have been taken should the laboratory reports be brought into the picture.

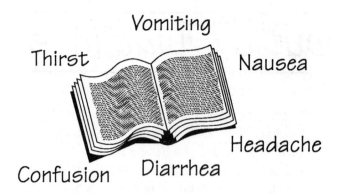

Vomiting
Thirst
Nausea
Headache
Confusion
Diarrhea

History taking will involve a search for volume loss, such as vomiting or diarrhea.

In a conscious patient symptoms may include thirst (which may be caused by water depletion or E.C.F. volume depletion), nausea (occurring in E.C.F. volume depletion) or headache and confusion (indicating I.C.F. volume changes).

Fluid Balance Charts

Time	In	Out

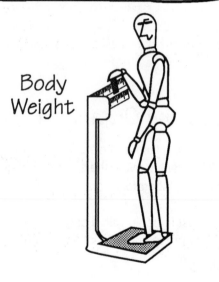

Body Weight

The patient's record may be helpful, and fluid balance charts are valuable. However, fluid charts can be misleading if they are not kept accurately.

Daily records of body weight are extremely useful as an index of changing body water, and they should always be consulted.

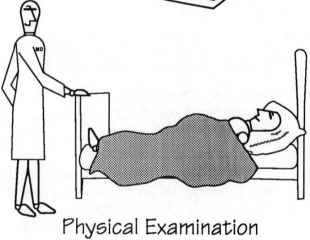

Physical Examination

Physical examination should be meticulous. Most of the physical signs that may be noted will relate to the E.C.F. compartment. It is important to remember that the I.C.F. is not readily accessible to clinical examination.

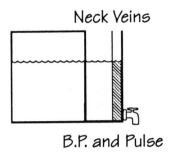

Neck Veins

B.P. and Pulse

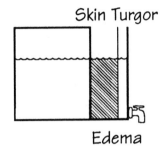

Skin Turgor

Edema

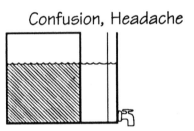

Confusion, Headache

Assessment of Volume

The plasma volume can be assessed by examining the jugular veins, checking the pulse rate and measuring the blood pressure. The blood pressure should be measured lying and sitting whenever possible since postural hypotension is an important sign of volume depletion.

The interstitial volume may be assessed by the presence or absence of edema, the degree of skin turgor and the state of the usually moist mucous membranes.

Changes of I.C.F. volume are less easy to detect and are usually reflected by headache, confusion and other evidence of disordered cerebral function. (review Chapter 5)

Fever

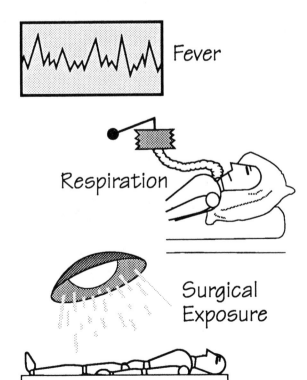

Respiration

Surgical Exposure

Losses of Body Water

It is important to remember that:

Losses of total body water are often underestimated. Major routes of increased loss include:

1) The skin: In fever with increased sweating and with high environmental temperatures.

2) The respiratory tract, with increased respiratory rate and loss of dead space in patients with endotracheal tubes.

3) Evaporative losses from operation sites. In prolonged surgical procedures where body cavities are exposed these may be very significant.

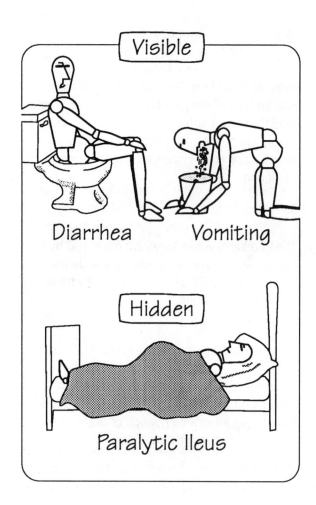

Visible

Diarrhea   Vomiting

Hidden

Paralytic Ileus

Losses of E.C.F.

It is important to remember that:

Losses of E.C.F. volume may be obvious as in the case of external losses due to vomiting or diarrhea.

But they may be hidden from view in a number of ways, for example:

1) Massive pooling of fluid may occur (sometimes after surgery) in a dilated and paralyzed intestine ("paralytic ileus"), or in the peritoneal cavity in peritonitis or if the bowel has an impaired blood supply.

2) Sudden increases of capillary permeability may cause the shift of a large volume of fluid out of the plasma compartment and into the interstitial space. This can occur in septicemic states.

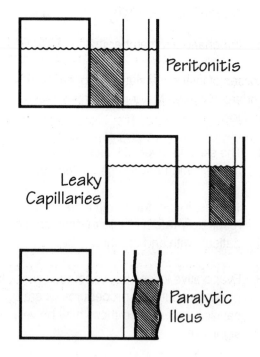

Peritonitis

Leaky Capillaries

Paralytic Ileus

The "Third" Space

In such situations total volume is not diminished, but shifts into some newly appearing "space" which (at least temporarily) is in communication with the E.C.F. It is as if the boundaries of the E.C.F. have suddenly expanded and as a result the normal volume does not fill all the space available. This is sometimes called the "third space" phenomenon.

Filling of such a "third space" can be a cause of all the signs of E.C.F. volume depletion, without obvious external loss. When such a space disappears (e.g. when paralytic ileus resolves) the volume may return rapidly into the E.C.F. and cause volume overload, particularly if renal function is impaired.

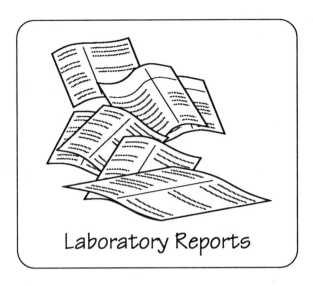

Laboratory Reports

Laboratory Tests

Only after a full assessment of the clinical background should the laboratory results be considered in detail.

Here are a few general rules about plasma electrolyte concentrations that may be helpful.

These are some of the more obvious changes seen in plasma electrolytes, and you should look for them. The list is not all inclusive, but will be a guide in handling the figures.

Plasma Sodium

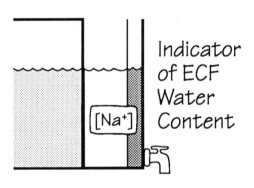

Indicator of ECF Water Content

The plasma sodium is an indicator of E.C.F. water content rather than E.C.F. sodium content. Profound E.C.F. volume depletion can occur with a normal plasma sodium because fluids lost by many routes are isotonic.

Before diagnosing a low plasma sodium as due to sodium depletion, make sure the patient has clinical evidence of E.C.F. volume depletion.

Plasma Potassium

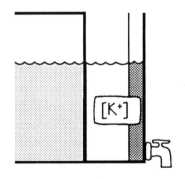

The plasma potassium will change either as a reflection of changes of total body potassium or of shifts of potassium into, or out of, the cells.

Changes of plasma potassium often reflect changes of pH status, or of blood sugar, rather than gains or losses of body potassium.

The Plasma Anion Gap

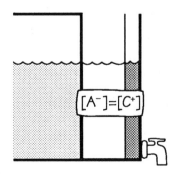

Plasma anions and cations will always be present in equal concentrations, but since not all anions are measured there will appear to be a gap between cations and anions. (Refer to Chapter 8).

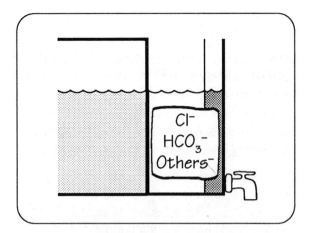

If the anion gap remains "constant" then changes in chloride and bicarbonate will go hand in hand. A low bicarbonate will cause a high chloride (hyperchloremic acidosis) but equally a high chloride will cause a low bicarbonate. Thus whether chloride or bicarbonate changes first, the other will show a reciprocal change.

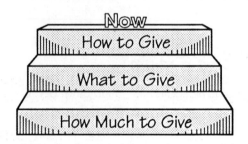

The Next Steps

Now that history and physical examination have been linked with laboratory data you can move on to the next steps:

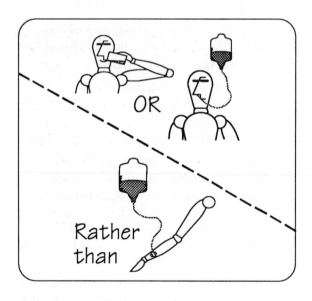

Which Route To Use

Whenever possible, fluid replacement should be administered by the normal physiologic route which is, of course, by mouth. It is surprising how often this basic rule is forgotten.

This is because modern equipment has made the intravenous route so easy to use; but it is important to remember that intravenous lines are a major source of in-hospital infection.

Other rarely used parenteral routes are subcutaneous or intraperitoneal infusions.

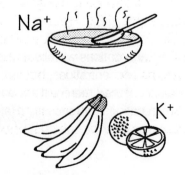

Electrolyte supplements can also be administered orally. This can be done using natural foods; soups are rich in sodium whilst many fruits and fruit juices contain potassium.

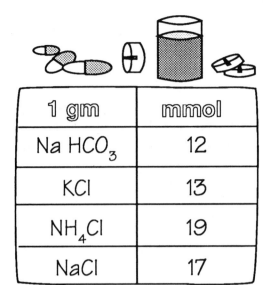

1 gm	mmol
Na HCO$_3$	12
KCl	13
NH$_4$Cl	19
NaCl	17

When supplements are added in artificial form it is more realistic to think in molar terms than in terms of weight. Thus 1 gram of sodium chloride contains 17 millimoles of sodium chloride whilst 1 gram of potassium chloride contains 13 millimoles of potassium chloride.

When intravenous (I.V.) fluid therapy has been decided upon, certain general principles determine the kind of fluid to be used.

What To Give

1) Water has to be given as "5% dextrose in water" since pure water would hemolyze the red cells as it enters the vein. Adding dextrose renders the water isotonic, but the dextrose is rapidly metabolized, leaving water.

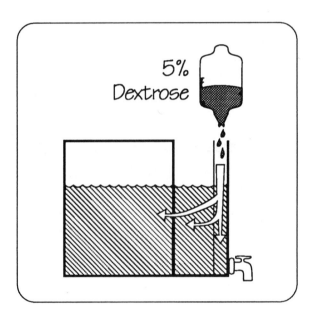

5% Dextrose

This will be distributed evenly throughout all body compartments and will contribute to both E.C.F. and I.C.F. The relative size of these compartments determines that two thirds of any water load will enter the I.C.F. and only one third will remain in the E.C.F. Thus three litres of 5% dextrose and water would theoretically be needed to expand the E.C.F. by only one litre. This fluid therefore is designed to replace deficits of total body water and not E.C.F. volume.

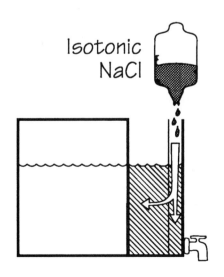

Isotonic NaCl

2) Isotonic sodium chloride will be distributed throughout the E.C.F. and will not enter the I.C.F. Such a solution is designed to replace deficits of E.C.F. volume. Thus 1 litre of isotonic sodium chloride will expand the E.C.F. by one litre; it will contribute to both plasma and interstitial compartments but because of their relative size, one litre of isotonic saline will theoretically only expand the plasma volume by one quarter of a litre.

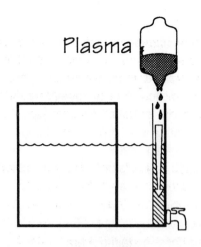

Plasma

3) Plasma, whole blood or "plasma expanders" are confined to the plasma volume and are designed to replace deficits in the volume of the plasma compartment only. Theoretically one litre of plasma will expand the plasma volume by one litre.

The risk of viral infection from pooled plasma has unfortunately limited its usefulness and plasma substitutes rather than plasma itself, are therefore often preferred.

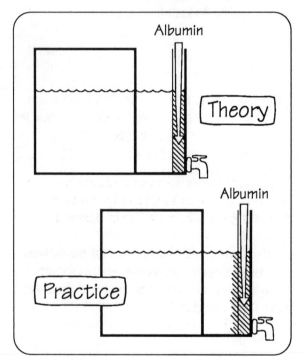

Albumin

Theory

Albumin

Practice

The precise distribution of fluids may not accord with theoretical ideals. Albumin, for example, is often considered a "plasma expander" when given intravenously, but in the long term probably becomes distributed throughout a much wider volume than that of plasma alone.

In the short term, however, theory and practice coincide well enough for albumin to function as a substitute for plasma.

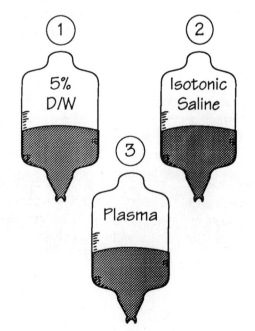

① 5% D/W

② Isotonic Saline

③ Plasma

For practical purposes therefore three intravenous fluids can form the basis of any volume replacement regimen. These fluids are

1) 5% dextrose in water

2) Isotonic sodium chloride

3) Plasma (or plasma substitute)

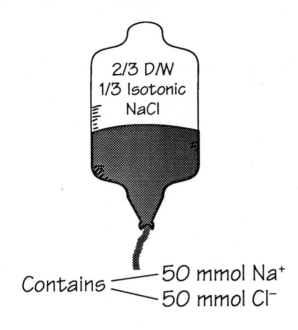

Contains — 50 mmol Na$^+$
— 50 mmol Cl$^-$

Many other intravenous solutions are available in containers suitable for immediate intravenous infusion. Many of them are widely used; in particular, mixtures of dextrose and saline such as "two thirds dextrose, one third isotonic saline".

A fluid such as this is useful in "maintenance" fluid replacement (see below) and is a convenience rather than a necessity. It is hypotonic, as far as the E.C.F. is concerned, and its uncritical use can be a cause of dilutional hyponatremia.

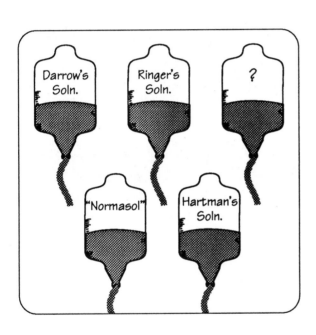

A number of more complex solutions is available and often sanctified by the term "physiological" which can be misleading.

They should be used only after careful thought and appropriate experience. Some of them have trade names which may give little clue to their exact composition.

Ringer's Lactate

Na$^+$	130 mmol/L
Cl$^-$	113 mmol/L
K$^+$	4 mmol/L
Ca^{2+}	3 mmol/L
Lactate	27 mmol/L

They include "balanced salt" solutions such as Ringer's-lactate solution. This solution contains potassium and calcium as well as lactate which is converted to bicarbonate by the liver.

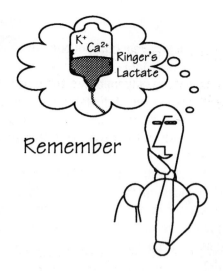

Remember

Such a fluid administered to a patient with lactic acidosis can, of course, be dangerous since failure to convert lactate to bicarbonate will make matters worse. In addition, the presence of potassium and calcium in the fluid is not indicated by its name and may be forgotten.

So with these "predesigned solutions" it is important before they are used to know (1) what they contain and (2) what their special risks may be.

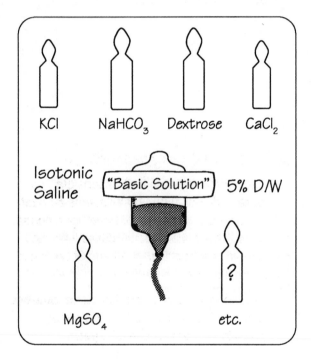

An alternative to such solutions is to use a "basic" fluid (5% dextrose or isotonic saline) and add concentrated solutions to it from prepacked ampoules.

The advantage of this is that each addition is made consciously (rather than automatically by a distant manufacturer) and that bicarbonate (which is easy to sterilize commercially in small containers) is available. Some of the more useful additives are shown here.

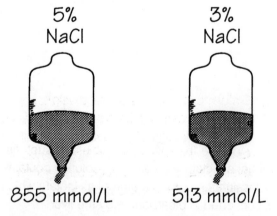

Only used in Acute Symptomatic Hyponatremia

A word about "hypertonic saline". It is only rarely indicated for severe and rapidly developing symptomatic hyponatremia. It is important to realize that it contains a great deal of sodium and chloride and should be used with great care.

Since most hyponatremic patients are edematous, (and therefore have already got an excess of body sodium), further sodium loading will increase the edema, and water restriction is the correct approach to most asymptomatic hyponatremic patients.

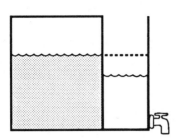

① Make up Losses that *have* ocurred

Then:

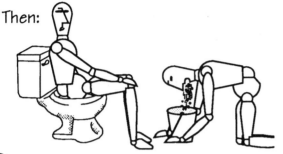

② Keep up with *Continuing* Losses

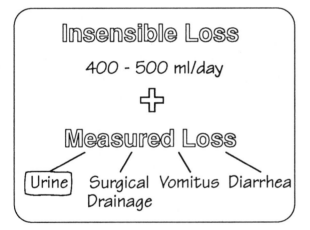

Insensible Loss

400 - 500 ml/day

✚

Measured Loss

Urine | Surgical Drainage | Vomitus | Diarrhea

To Measure Fluid Gain or Loss

Body Weight

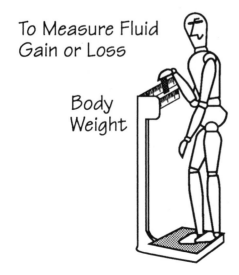

How Much To Give

In any fluid therapy there are two main objectives.

1) To make up the losses that have already occurred.

2) To keep up with the losses that are occurring whilst fluids are being given.

Some general rules may be of help.

1) Basic unmeasurable and "insensible" losses that will occur in all patients amount to 400-500 millilitres in 24 hours for a normal adult. This is made up of losses from the skin, the lungs and a small amount of water in normal feces.

As mentioned earlier, both of these routes of loss may increase greatly in abnormal conditions or environmental stress.

2) Serial measurements of body weight are extremely useful indicators of loss or gain of fluid. Knowledge of the patient's weight before sustaining a volume loss may be available and will be a good guide to the volume of fluid needed to replace the loss.

Correction Results In

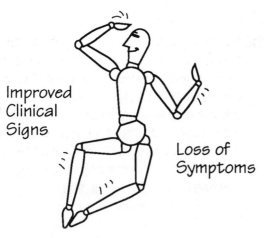

Improved Clinical Signs

Loss of Symptoms

3) The loss of symptoms such as thirst and nausea will be a guide towards the degree of correction of volume loss that has been achieved.

Similarly, careful clinical assessment will indicate such things as the return of blood pressure and pulse to normal. The appearance of moist sounds in previously dry lung bases indicates that volume requirements have been over-corrected.

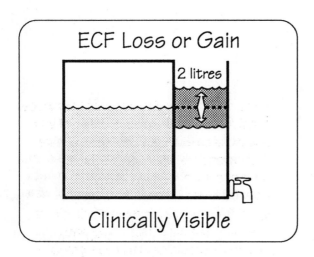

ECF Loss or Gain

2 litres

Clinically Visible

4) In order to show clear signs of volume depletion or overload an adult is usually at least two litres up or down as far as the E.C.F. volume is concerned. Often, of course, the size of the deficit, or excess, will be much greater than this.

Smaller losses will produce more subtle clinical signs which may easily be missed.

I.V. Fluids Safer, If:

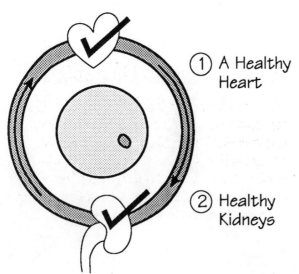

① A Healthy Heart

② Healthy Kidneys

5) As clinicians, our margin of safety is usually wide because the body can manipulate almost any parenteral load provided the kidneys and heart function normally.

But, in patients with known cardiac or renal disease, or in the older patient whose cardiac and renal reserves may be limited, much more care must be taken with intravenous fluids.

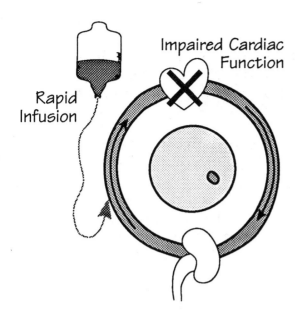

6) The rate of infusion is as important as the total amount that is given. Thus the rapid infusion of volume into the venous side of the circulation in a patient with heart disease may temporarily exceed the ability of the heart to distribute the added volume and pulmonary edema may develop before a deficit of E.C.F. volume has been fully corrected.

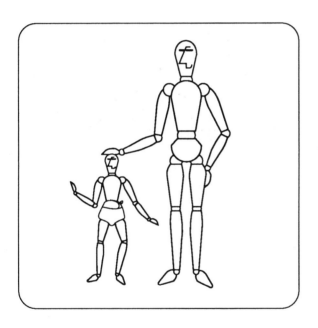

7) Variations of body size and weight must be considered. Fluid replacement in infants and small children requires special care and experience, although the same general principles apply at any age. Reference was made in Chapter 3 to special factors that occur in small infants. The management of major fluid and electrolyte problems in this age group requires specialized skill and experience.

A Note About Diuretics

Diuretics are important agents which act upon the renal tubule to increase urine flow. They find their major therapeutic role in states of sodium and water retention associated with edema. They can be divided into the three types shown here; transport inhibitors are by far the most important in a clinical setting.

① Osmotic Diuretics

② ADH Antagonists

③ Transport Inhibitors

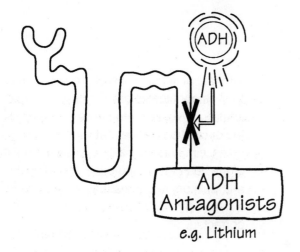

ADH Antagonists

e.g. Lithium

Some agents block the action of ADH upon the collecting duct and thus produce loss of water without significant loss of solute.

They include lithium carbonate and demeclocycline and have a minor clinical role as agents to promote water excretion in states of inappropriate ADH release.

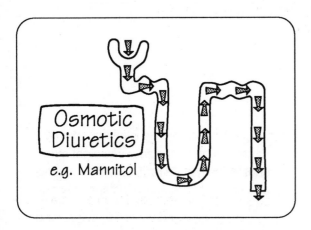

Osmotic Diuretics

e.g. Mannitol

Some agents act as diuretics by being non-absorbable solutes which, once filtered, move through the tubule without any absorption and thus generate osmotic effects which keep water and solutes within the tubule.

In diabetes mellitus the high filtered concentrations of glucose can act in this way.

Mannitol is sometimes used clinically to promote rapid urine flow, and finds a place in the management of impending acute renal failure.

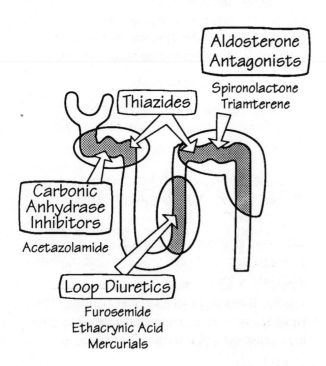

Aldosterone Antagonists

Spironolactone
Triamterene

Thiazides

Carbonic Anhydrase Inhibitors

Acetazolamide

Loop Diuretics

Furosemide
Ethacrynic Acid
Mercurials

The major diuretics are all inhibitors of ionic transport processes at one or more sites in the tubule. Their precise mode of action is not always well understood, but some general comments can be made.

i) Carbonic anhydrase inhibitors block the generation of bicarbonate and hydrogen ions in the tubule, and limit sodium reabsorption by limiting the availability of hydrogen ion for exchange.

ii) Diuretics acting in the loop of Henle interfere with chloride and sodium transport and secondarily interfere with urine concentration.

iii) Diuretics acting on the distal tubule include antagonists of aldosterone and block sodium reabsorption whilst encouraging retention of potassium.

iv) Some diuretics (like the thiazides) seem to act at more than one site and their action is incompletely understood.

Because these inhibitors are both potent and non-selective they can produce side effects by disturbing physiologic regulation. For example, except for the aldosterone antagonists, they all block reabsorption of potassium as well as sodium, which is why potassium supplements may be needed with these drugs.

These side effects can be very important and the use of diuretics demands knowledge of their risks as well as benefits.

Some Specific Problems

1) Maintenance Fluids

"Maintenance" fluid therapy for an average normal adult, with normal renal function, who cannot take orally for a few days can be based on the following general requirements.

Water   2000 millilitres per day
Sodium   75-100 millimoles per day
Potassium   50 millimoles per day

This can be provided by giving

i)   1500 millilitres of 5% dextrose and 500 millilitres of isotonic sodium chloride with added potassium.
     or
ii) 2000 millilitres of "2/3 5% dextrose, 1/3 isotonic sodium chloride" with added potassium.

With healthy kidneys the limits of error are wide, but with coincident kidney disease this regime must be modified.

Additional calories can be added by using 10% dextrose, but "maintenance fluids" for a few days does not equate with "total parenteral nutrition".

Maintenance Fluids

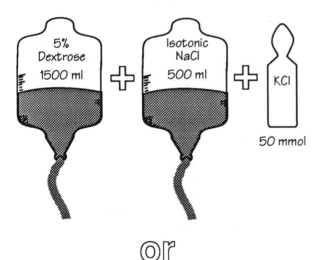

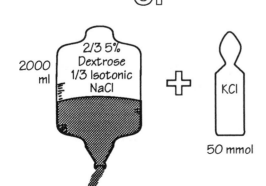

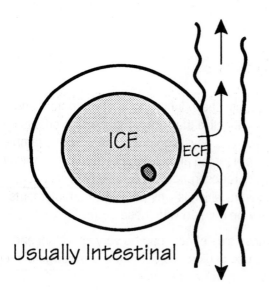

Usually Intestinal

2) E.C.F. Loss

The common site for E.C.F. fluid losses is from the intestine. Such losses should be replaced by isotonic sodium chloride as a first step. Appropriate additions to this fluid will be dictated by the site of loss. With the exception of colonic diarrheal fluid, all intestinal losses are effectively isotonic with the E.C.F.

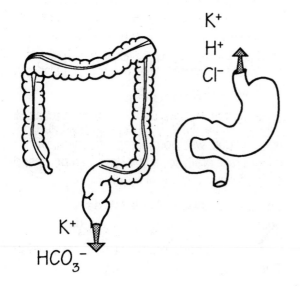

K^+

H^+

Cl^-

K^+

HCO_3^-

Vomiting will be associated with hypokalemia, hypochloremia and alkalosis as well as volume depletion.

Severe diarrhea will be associated with hypokalemia and sometimes hyperchloremic acidosis as well as volume depletion.

Colonic diarrhea will lead to hypotonic fluid losses.

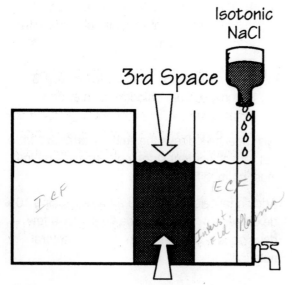

Isotonic NaCl

3rd Space

In general, a "third space" may be considered as being in communication with the E.C.F. and replacement therapy should also be with isotonic sodium chloride as a first step.

160

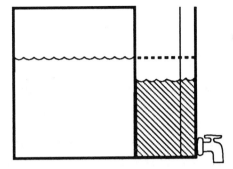

Massive Losses of Plasma Colloids and ECF

3) Burns

Burns are a special problem and involve massive loss of plasma colloids as well as E.C.F. Fluid replacement in such patients is the key to initial survival and the amounts of fluid required may be very large. Detailed texts should be consulted for methods of calculation of fluid needs.

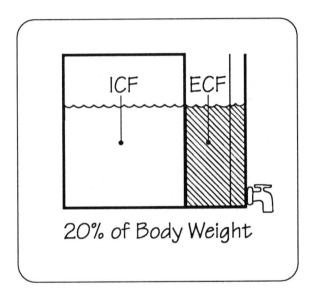

20% of Body Weight

4) Bicarbonate Therapy

Sometimes, in a severe metabolic acidosis, bicarbonate is infused intravenously to correct extracellular pH. Deciding how much bicarbonate to give is an example of some of the problems inherent in replacing one specific E.C.F. constituent.

Knowing that the total E.C.F. volume in an adult is 20% of body weight and knowing that the "normal" bicarbonate concentration in the E.C.F. is 25 millimoles per litre, it is obviously a simple matter to calculate the deficit of bicarbonate in the E.C.F. in this way:

Deficit = (25 - measured plasma bicarbonate) x 20% of body weight

Bicarbonate Distribution

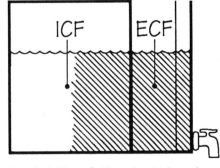

40-50% of Body Weight

Unfortunately it is not that simple because

i)   The true volume of distribution for bicarbonate exceeds the E.C.F. volume and probably approximates two-thirds of total body water (i.e. 40-50% of body weight) or even more.

ii)   Rapid and complete replacement of a deficit can produce dangerous side effects. (See below)

An Example

Measured Plasma HCO_3^-	11 mmol/L
"Normal" Plasma $[HCO_3^-]$	25 mmol/L
Deficit	25-11=14mmol/L
Half of Deficit	14/5=7mmol/L

Body Weight	75 Kg
ECF Volume	20% of 75=15L

Amount of HCO_3^- given will
be 15 x 17 = 105 mmol

So - it is usually considered practical wisdom to attempt to correct the measured E.C.F. bicarbonate concentration only half way to its "normal" value of 25 millimoles per litre and to assume a volume of distribution that approximates the E.C.F. volume. This is a first step in replacement and ensures that it will deliberately fall well short of complete correction. The amount given will probably be no more than half the actual deficit.

Having given this amount of bicarbonate a reassessment of clinical and laboratory data will determine the next step.

Severe degrees of metabolic acidosis may demand very large amounts of bicarbonate, but overenthusiastic treatment can have risks.

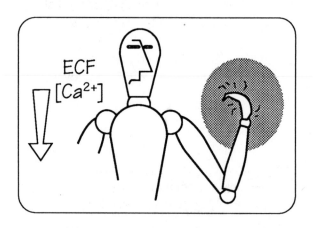

a) Too much, too quickly, may produce tetany or convulsions by lowering ionized calcium concentration. (See Chapter 10)

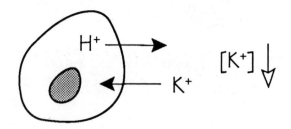

b) It may also produce hypokalemia as potassium ions return to the cells in exchange for hydrogen ions that have been buffered in the I.C.F. (See Chapter 9)

162

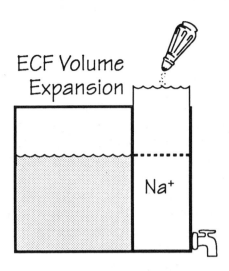

ECF Volume
Expansion

Na⁺

c) The bicarbonate must be given as a sodium salt and the sodium may lead to over-expansion of the E.C.F. volume. (See Chapter 6)

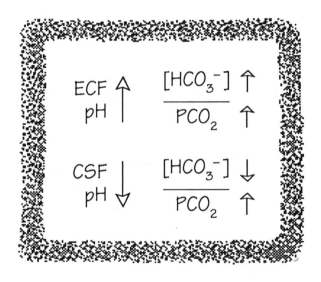

$$ECF\ pH \uparrow \qquad \frac{[HCO_3^-] \uparrow}{PCO_2 \uparrow}$$

$$CSF\ pH \downarrow \qquad \frac{[HCO_3^-] \downarrow}{PCO_2 \uparrow}$$

d) As bicarbonate concentrations rise, so the pH rises and the PCO_2 will also rise. But the PCO_2 rapidly equilibrates with the cerebrospinal fluid (C.S.F.) whilst the bicarbonate only slowly crosses the barrier between the E.C.F. and the C.S.F. Thus in the C.S.F. the PCO_2 rises but the bicarbonate remains relatively constant. As a result, a rising pH in the E.C.F. may occur but a further fall in pH will occur in the C.S.F. leading to major disturbances of brain function such as convulsions.

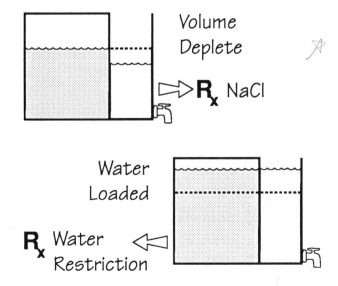

Volume
Deplete

R_x NaCl

Water
Loaded

R_x Water
Restriction

5) Treating Hyponatremia

The two basic general rules are:

a) If the patient is volume deplete, they need sodium chloride. If given intravenously, isotonic saline is appropriate.

b) If volume replete (and usually with obvious edema), they need water restriction because they are water loaded.

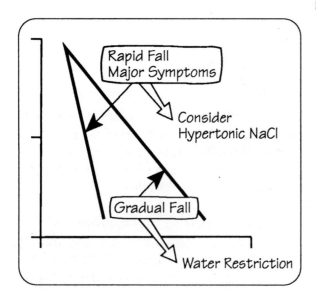

Severe, rapidly developing symptomatic hyponatremia leads to acute cell swelling and may produce neurological disturbances and convulsions. When this occurs a rapid correction of the plasma sodium may seem desirable. Hypertonic NaCl can be used (usually as "3% saline", which contains 513 mmol of NaCl/L).

This is only rarely indicated and has the risk that rapid reversal of hypotonicity may lead to further neurological damage including "central pontine myelinolysis" which can be lethal.

If hypertonic saline is used, conventional wisdom suggests that the rate of increase of plasma sodium should not exceed 0.5 mmol/L/hour.

6) Treating Hypernatremia

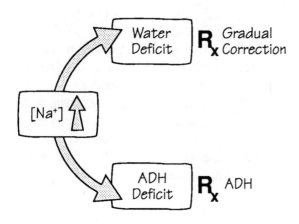

Rapid correction of hypernatremia can also lead to rapid shifts of water into brain cells. This can result in brain swelling with convulsions and severe cerebral damage. Correction should be achieved by giving free water by mouth where possible. If free water is given intravenously (usually as 5% dextrose and water) correction should be gradual and not abrupt, with similar concerns to those involved in rapid correction of hyponatremia.

Clearly hypernatremia due to ADH deficiency should be treated by ADH administration as well as the provision of free water.

7) Treating Hyperkalemia

Because of the toxic effect of potassium on the heart, hyperkalemia may be an acute medical emergency. (See Chapter 9).

Management of hyperkalemia can involve three approaches; the choice of which to use depends upon the urgency of the clinical situation.

a) The toxic effect of potassium on the heart can be blocked using the antagonistic effect of calcium. This does not alter the plasma potassium concentration but reverses (temporarily) its toxic effect on the heart. Intravenous calcium gluconate, or in an acute emergency calcium chloride, may be used.

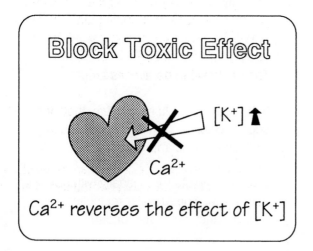

Push K⁺ into the Cells

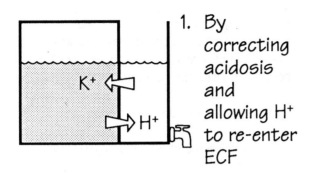

1. By correcting acidosis and allowing H⁺ to re-enter ECF

b) The potassium can be pushed back into the I.C.F. This can be done by rapid correction of coincident acidosis, in which case hydrogen ions begin to leave the cells and potassium re-enters them.

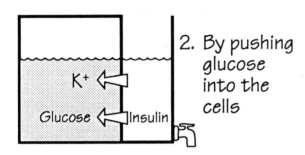

2. By pushing glucose into the cells

The same effect can be achieved by infusing glucose and insulin. Insulin pushes glucose into the cell and results in co-transport of potassium with the glucose.

In diabetic ketoacidosis potassium will re-enter the cells rapidly as insulin is administered, an example of the mechanism linking potassium and glucose transport.

Remove K⁺ from E.C.F.

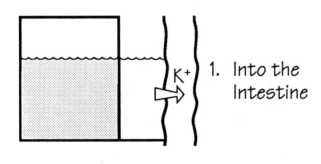

1. Into the Intestine

c) Potassium can be removed from the E.C.F. directly. One way of doing this is to lose it into the intestine by inducing diarrhea or by using ion-exchange resins that will fix potassium in exchange for some other cation (usually sodium or calcium).

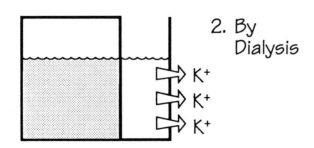

2. By Dialysis

Alternatively artificial dialysis can be used either by peritoneal lavage or the use of an extra-corporeal dialyzer.

Replacement

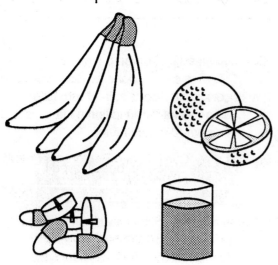

8) Treating Hypokalemia

Hypokalemia is seldom an acute, life-threatening situation and is often associated with a shift of hydrogen ions as well as actual potassium loss. (See Chapter 9)

Treatment of hypokalemia includes

a) Correcting the cause of potassium loss

b) Correcting the cause of alkalosis and then

c) Prescribing potassium supplements whenever possible by the oral route, since hypokalemia is seldom an emergency.

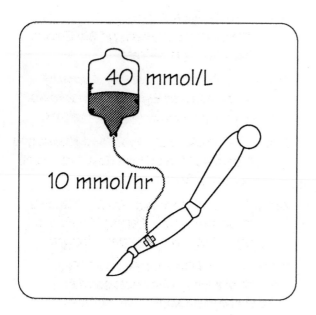

When intravenous potassium is used a note of caution is in order.

Intravenous potassium is safe if used in low concentrations and at slow rates of infusion.

Concentrations above 40 millimoles per litre and infusion rates above 10 millimoles per hour should be avoided accept in special circumstances.

Concentrations above 60 millimoles per litre and infusion rates above 40 millimoles per hour should never be used without experience and careful monitoring. Such concentrations should not be given for more than 2 or 3 hours without careful reassessment.

Further Reading

Of Historic Interest

Pitts R.F. (1968) *"Physiology of the Kidney and Body Fluids"* 2nd Edition. Year Book Publishers, Chicago.

Smith H.W. (1959) *"From Fish to Philosopher"*. Ciba Edition with permission of Little, Brown and Company, Boston.

Welt L.G. (1959) *"Clinical Disorders of Hydration and Acid Base Equilibrium"* 2nd Edition. Little, Brown and Company, Boston.

General Resources

Brenner B.M. and Rector F.C. (1990) Eds. *"The Kidney"* 4th Edition. W.B. Saunders, Philadelphia.

Brenner B.M., Coe F.L. and Rector F.C. (1987). *"Renal Physiology in Health and Disease"*. W.B. Saunders, Philadelphia.

Halperin M.L. and Goldstein M.B. (1988). *"Fluid, Electrolyte and Acid-Base Emergencies"*. W.B. Saunders, Philadelphia.

Kokko J.P. and Tannen R.L. (1990) Eds. *"Fluid and Electrolytes"* 2nd Edition. W.B. Saunders, Philadelphia.

Leaf A. and Cotran R.S. (1985). *"Renal Pathophysiology"* 3rd Edition. Oxford University Press.

Rose B.D. (1989). *"Clinical Physiology of Acid-Base and Electrolyte Disorders"* 3rd. Edition. McGraw Hill, New York.

Schrier R.W. (1986) Ed. *"Renal and Electrolyte Disorders"* 3rd Edition. Little, Brown and Company, Boston.

Schrier R.W. and Gottschalk C.W. (1988) Eds. *"Diseases of the Kidney"* 4th Edition. Little, Brown and Company, Boston.

Seldin D.W. and Giebisch G. (1985) Eds. *"The Kidney - Physiology and Pathophysiology"*. Raven Press, New York.

Smith E.K.M. (1987). *"Renal Disease - A Conceptual Approach"*. Churchill Livingstone, New York.

Vander A.J. (1991).*"Renal Physiology"* 4th Edition. McGraw-Hill, New York.

Index of Topics

Index of Topics

Index of Topics

Index of Topics

Index of Topics